SUZANNE BYRD

Unmasking Autism in Women

Understanding the Female Spectrum

Contents

1

Introduction – The Unseen Spectrum

Autism has long been a subject of fascination, misunderstanding, and evolving research. Yet, much of the discourse has historically centered on a narrow, male-oriented view of the condition, leaving many women and girls in the shadows. In this opening chapter, we set the stage for a deeper exploration of autism as it appears in women—a journey that uncovers the subtle presentations and masking behaviors that too often lead to misdiagnosis and misunderstanding.

A Call for Recognition

For decades, autism research and societal narratives have painted a picture of the condition that fails to capture its rich diversity. Seminal works like Steve Silberman's *NeuroTribes: The Legacy of Autism* have done much to broaden our understanding of autism's history and impact. However, even these comprehensive studies have only recently begun to address the nuances of autism in women. This book is a response to that gap—a call to acknowledge and celebrate the unique experiences of autistic women, whether they are formally diagnosed or self-identified.

Autistic women often find themselves on a diagnostic roller coaster.

Many navigate a labyrinth of misdiagnoses, as their behaviors and challenges do not fit the stereotypical autism profile. Instead of the overt symptoms traditionally associated with autism, these women display a "female autism phenotype," characterized by subtler social difficulties, a propensity for masking, and an intense internal world that remains largely hidden from public view. The narrative of their lives, until now, has been largely unwritten in mainstream literature and clinical research.

The Landscape of Misdiagnosis

The journey to an accurate diagnosis for many autistic women is fraught with hurdles. Cultural expectations and gender norms have long influenced the way behaviors are interpreted. For example, traits like shyness, empathy, or an intense focus on specific interests—common among autistic women—are often seen as quirks or even strengths rather than signs of a neurodevelopmental difference. This can lead to an under-recognition of the condition, leaving many to suffer in silence.

Books such as Liane Holliday Willey's *Pretending to be Normal: Living with Asperger's Syndrome* offer invaluable insights into the experience of masking—where autistic individuals consciously or unconsciously mimic neurotypical behaviors to fit in. While Willey's work primarily focuses on her personal journey, its themes resonate deeply with the experiences of many women on the spectrum. The pressure to conform to societal expectations can be overwhelming, often resulting in chronic stress, anxiety, and a profound sense of isolation.

Unmasking the Hidden Self

At the heart of this book lies the concept of masking—the deliberate act of hiding one's true self to avoid judgment or rejection. Masking is not merely a surface behavior; it is a survival mechanism born out of a lifetime of having to navigate environments that are not designed for neurodivergent minds. Autistic women, in particular, are adept at this performance. They learn to observe, imitate, and sometimes even overcompensate in social settings, often at great personal cost.

In *The Reason I Jump*, celebrated autistic author Naoki Higashida provides a window into the inner workings of an autistic mind. Although his perspective is not gender-specific, his descriptions of the sensory and emotional experiences of autism are universally resonant. For women, the stakes of masking are higher because their ability to adapt often leads to their struggles being overlooked. The energy expended in this constant performance can lead to burnout and a fragmented sense of identity.

The Intersection of Gender and Neurodiversity

The intersection of gender and neurodiversity creates a complex tapestry of challenges and strengths. Society's expectations of femininity—such as emotional expressiveness, sociability, and nurturing behaviors—can both obscure and exacerbate the difficulties autistic women face. When an autistic woman conforms to these expectations, her challenges might be minimized or misinterpreted; when she does not, she risks harsh judgment for deviating from the norm.

Drawing on research and personal accounts from a variety of sources, including works like Tony Attwood's *The Complete Guide to Asperger's Syndrome*, we begin to see a pattern. Autistic women often develop sophisticated coping strategies that allow them to "blend in," but these strategies can mask underlying struggles that require attention. The societal imperative to appear "normal" can force women to trade authenticity for acceptance—a choice that exacts a heavy emotional toll.

Navigating a World of Stereotypes

Stereotypes about autism have long been rooted in outdated research and societal misconceptions. Historically, autism was seen as a condition predominantly affecting boys, a perspective that influenced diagnostic criteria and treatment approaches for decades. This skewed view not only marginalized women but also perpetuated a cycle of underdiagnosis and misinterpretation.

In recent years, a growing body of literature has begun to dismantle these stereotypes. Books like *Women and Autism Spectrum Disorder* by Sarah Hendrickx and colleagues have shed light on the distinct ways autism manifests in women, highlighting the need for tailored approaches in both research and practice. By challenging long-held assumptions, these works have paved the way for a more inclusive understanding of autism—a movement that this book proudly continues.

The Personal and the Universal

While the statistics and research underscore the broader trends, the heart of this exploration lies in personal stories—the lived experiences of autistic women who have long felt unseen and unheard. Their narratives are a powerful reminder that behind every clinical label is a human being with hopes, dreams, and struggles. Throughout this book, we will share voices from across the spectrum, each contributing a unique perspective to the collective understanding of female autism.

For instance, consider the story of Maya, a young woman whose journey to an accurate diagnosis was marked by years of self-doubt and societal pressure. Despite her academic achievements and creative talents, Maya was frequently told that her sensitivity and introspection were simply signs of a "female temperament." It wasn't until she encountered a clinician who recognized the nuances of the female autism phenotype that her true self began to emerge. Maya's story is echoed in many lives, illustrating the profound impact of delayed recognition and the transformative power of self-acceptance.

The Importance of Understanding

Understanding the female autism phenotype is not just a matter of academic interest—it is a crucial step towards creating a more supportive and inclusive society. By recognizing the unique challenges faced by autistic women, we can begin to dismantle the barriers that prevent them from accessing the resources and support they need. This understanding fosters empathy, encourages early intervention, and ultimately leads to better outcomes for individuals and families alike.

The implications extend beyond the realm of personal well-being. As more autistic women come forward with their stories, there is a growing movement to reshape public policy, improve educational practices, and create work environments that accommodate neurodiversity. The conversation is shifting from one of deficit to one of difference— recognizing that what has been traditionally labeled as "symptoms" may, in fact, be unique strengths waiting to be harnessed.

A Roadmap for the Journey Ahead

In the chapters that follow, we will delve into the multifaceted world of female autism. We will explore the biological, psychological, and social dimensions of the condition, drawing on the latest research as well as firsthand accounts from autistic women and experts in the field. Each chapter is designed to build a comprehensive picture of what it means to live as an autistic woman in a world that often fails to see beyond the surface.

Our journey will take us through the historical evolution of autism diagnosis, the intricacies of masking and its consequences, and the transformative impact of self-advocacy. We will examine the challenges of relationships, mental health, and career success, while also highlighting the resilience and creativity that many autistic women embody. Along the way, we will reference a range of influential works—from Tony Attwood's clinical insights to the personal narratives found in Liane Holliday Willey's writings—to provide a well-rounded perspective on the subject.

Setting the Stage for Empowerment

At its core, *Unmasking Autism in Women: Understanding the Female Spectrum* is about empowerment. It is an invitation for autistic women to reclaim their narratives and celebrate the complexity of their identities. The act of unmasking is not about shedding one's protective behaviors overnight; it is about embracing authenticity, understanding one's strengths, and building a community that values diversity in all its forms.

This book is dedicated to every woman who has ever felt pressured to hide her true self, every parent who has struggled to understand their child's unique needs, and every clinician who is committed to evolving their practice to better serve a diverse population. Through research, reflection, and personal stories, we aim to create a resource that not only educates but also inspires hope and fosters a sense of belonging.

Embracing a New Narrative

The journey toward understanding and acceptance begins with a single step: acknowledging that the narrative of autism must expand to include all voices, especially those that have been marginalized for too long. In redefining autism through the lens of female experience, we are not erasing the challenges that exist; rather, we are enriching the conversation by adding depth and nuance.

As you read through this book, you will encounter ideas that challenge conventional wisdom, inspiring a reevaluation of what it means to be autistic. We invite you to approach this material with an open mind and a compassionate heart, recognizing that every experience is valid and every story is worth telling.

In conclusion, this opening chapter has set the stage for an exploration of the unseen spectrum—the hidden facets of autism in women that have been obscured by stereotypes and misdiagnosis. By drawing on a diverse range of sources and personal narratives, we aim to illuminate the path toward greater understanding and support. The journey ahead is both a personal and collective one, and it is our hope that through these pages, you will find validation, insight, and the courage to unmask your true self.

NeuroTribes by Steve Silberman, *Pretending to be Normal* by Liane Holliday Willey, and Tony Attwood's extensive work on autism have all contributed to the evolving conversation around neurodiversity. Their insights serve as important waypoints on our journey, reminding us that every story—no matter how quietly told—has the power to change lives. As we move forward, let us remember that understanding is the first step towards acceptance and that the unseen spectrum deserves to be seen in all its complexity.

By redefining the narrative around autism in women, we not only foster a deeper understanding of the condition but also create a future where differences are celebrated rather than hidden. Welcome to a new chapter in the ongoing story of neurodiversity—a journey toward unmasking the truth, embracing authenticity, and ultimately, finding strength in being exactly who we are.

This chapter lays the foundation for the rest of the book. It challenges long-standing stereotypes, provides a historical context, and introduces the concept of masking as a survival mechanism. With references to influential works in the field, it aims to validate the lived experiences of autistic women and invite a more inclusive conversation. As you continue reading, you will gain further insights into the multifaceted nature of autism and discover practical ways to navigate a world that is slowly learning to understand and celebrate neurodiversity.

2

Defining Autism in the Context of Women

Understanding autism in women begins with a fundamental redefinition of the condition itself—one that moves beyond traditional, male-centric models to embrace a more nuanced view. In this chapter, we delve into what autism means when seen through the lens of femininity. We explore the broad spectrum of behaviors and experiences, discuss how gender influences both the manifestation and perception of autism, and draw on insights from seminal works in the field.

Rethinking Autism: A Broader Definition

Autism, historically defined by a set of observable behaviors, is now recognized as a complex neurodevelopmental condition that affects social communication, sensory processing, and executive functioning. Classic texts such as *NeuroTribes: The Legacy of Autism* by Steve Silberman have reshaped our understanding by illustrating that autism is not a single, homogenous condition but a spectrum with diverse presentations and strengths. Silberman's work underscores that the variability within autism calls for a more inclusive framework—one that accounts for subtle differences, particularly those evident in women.

Traditional diagnostic models have focused on traits that are more apparent in males: overt social challenges, repetitive behaviors, and difficulties with nonverbal communication. Yet, these criteria often miss the nuanced ways autism can present in women. While the core features of autism remain—differences in social interaction, communication, and sensory processing—the expression of these traits can be moderated by social expectations and learned behaviors. This shift in perspective is essential to appreciate the female experience of autism.

The Female Autism Phenotype: Unique Characteristics

A growing body of research has identified what many refer to as the "female autism phenotype." This concept encompasses the idea that autistic women may exhibit a different profile of behaviors compared to their male counterparts. Books like *Pretending to be Normal: Living with Asperger's Syndrome* by Liane Holliday Willey provide early insights into these differences, describing how many autistic women develop sophisticated coping mechanisms to navigate social situations. Instead of the overtly rigid behaviors often associated with autism, women may display more subtle forms of social communication challenges and emotional dysregulation.

Autistic women are often adept at "masking" their difficulties. Masking involves the conscious or unconscious effort to hide traits that might be perceived as socially unacceptable. This can include mimicking neurotypical behaviors, rehearsing conversational responses, and suppressing natural reactions. While these strategies may help in certain social contexts, they come at a significant personal cost. The effort required to maintain a façade often results in heightened stress, anxiety, and eventually, burnout. Tony Attwood's *The Complete Guide to Asperger's Syndrome* discusses similar themes, noting that the survival strategies employed by autistic individuals can be both a blessing and a curse—helpful in the short term yet potentially damaging to long-term mental health.

The female autism phenotype is characterized not just by masking but also by the internalization of struggles. Whereas men might externalize their challenges through disruptive behavior, autistic women often internalize feelings of inadequacy, leading to conditions such as anxiety and depression. This internalization is compounded by societal expectations that encourage women to be socially adept and emotionally expressive. When autistic women fail to meet these expectations, they are more likely to be blamed for their perceived shortcomings rather than understood as experiencing a neurodevelopmental difference.

The Spectrum: Understanding Variability

Autism is often described as a "spectrum" because it encompasses a wide range of abilities and challenges. The recognition of this variability has been a major milestone in autism research. The concept of neuro-diversity, which views neurological differences as natural variations rather than deficits, has been influential in shifting public perception. However, while neurodiversity celebrates differences, it also reminds us that each individual's experience is unique—especially when gender factors into the equation.

In women, the spectrum may manifest in less stereotypical ways. For instance, an autistic woman might have a deep interest in literature, art, or animals—a focus that, in another context, might be celebrated as a passion rather than seen as a restrictive interest. This recontextual-ization is crucial because it shifts the focus from what autistic women "lack" to what they can offer. Instead of viewing certain traits solely as symptoms, we begin to see them as expressions of individuality. As Silberman emphasizes in *NeuroTribes*, the diversity within the autism spectrum is a strength that enriches society when properly understood and supported.

Gender Roles and Social Conditioning

The influence of gender roles on the presentation of autism in women cannot be overstated. Society often imposes strict norms on behavior, particularly for women. From a young age, girls are socialized to be caring, empathetic, and communicative. These expectations can compel autistic girls and women to overcompensate for their social challenges. They learn to mimic the behaviors of their neurotypical peers, even when doing so conflicts with their natural inclinations.

Books such as *Women and Autism Spectrum Disorder* by Sarah Hendrickx and colleagues have highlighted how these social pressures affect diagnosis and self-perception. Autistic women are frequently misunderstood because their behaviors, while different, often align with socially acceptable female roles. For example, a strong preference for routine and detailed focus on specific interests might be misinterpreted as meticulousness or dedication—qualities that are often valued in women. Yet, beneath this veneer of normalcy, many women are battling sensory overload, social exhaustion, and the internal pain of not fitting neatly into prescribed roles.

This conflict between internal experience and external expectation is a recurring theme in the literature. Liane Holliday Willey's accounts in *Pretending to be Normal* illustrate how the pressure to conform can lead to a life of hidden distress. Many autistic women feel trapped between two worlds: one in which they are expected to perform a version of normalcy and another where their true selves, with all their complexities, remain unacknowledged.

The Diagnostic Challenge: Bridging the Gap

A significant barrier to understanding autism in women is the diagnostic framework itself. Many of the criteria used to diagnose autism were developed based on studies predominantly involving boys. As a result, these criteria may not fully capture the experiences of autistic girls and women. This diagnostic gap has led to numerous cases where autistic women are misdiagnosed with conditions such as anxiety, depression, or even borderline personality disorder. In some cases, the underlying autism is only recognized later in life, often after years of struggling to fit into a world that does not accommodate their needs.

The work of Tony Attwood, particularly in *The Complete Guide to Asperger's Syndrome*, has been instrumental in highlighting the need for more gender-sensitive diagnostic tools. Attwood points out that while the core challenges of autism are universal, the ways in which these challenges manifest can be deeply influenced by gender. For instance, while repetitive behaviors and special interests are common in autism, the interests pursued by autistic women may be more socially acceptable and therefore less likely to be flagged as atypical. This nuance necessitates a rethinking of diagnostic approaches to ensure that women receive the recognition and support they deserve.

Efforts to refine diagnostic criteria have begun to emerge, driven in part by the personal testimonies of autistic women who have experienced misdiagnosis firsthand. These voices, along with academic research, are gradually shifting the narrative towards a more inclusive understanding. As diagnostic practices evolve, they hold the promise of better identifying autistic women earlier in life, thereby opening the door to timely interventions and support.

Embracing Neurodiversity: A New Lens for Understanding

Central to redefining autism in the context of women is the broader concept of neurodiversity. Neurodiversity challenges the idea of "normalcy" and celebrates the natural variations in human brain function. It asserts that neurological differences, such as autism, should be recognized as a valuable part of human diversity rather than pathologized. This perspective is particularly liberating for autistic women, who have long been pressured to conform to narrow definitions of what it means to be "normal."

Books like *NeuroTribes* have been at the forefront of the neurodiversity movement, arguing that embracing neurological differences can lead to a more innovative and compassionate society. By applying this framework to the female autism phenotype, we can begin to appreciate the strengths and talents that often accompany these differences. Autistic women frequently possess exceptional attention to detail, creative problem-solving skills, and the ability to think outside conventional boundaries— qualities that are increasingly recognized as assets in a variety of fields.

Adopting a neurodiversity perspective also shifts the conversation from one of deficit to one of difference. Instead of focusing solely on the challenges that autistic women face, we can also celebrate their contributions and the unique insights they bring to the table. This holistic view is essential for fostering environments—whether in education, employment, or social settings—that accommodate a wider range of experiences and talents.

The Role of Self-Identity and Empowerment

A critical aspect of understanding autism in women is the interplay between self-identity and societal expectations. Autistic women often find themselves in a constant battle between embracing their true selves and conforming to external pressures. This struggle can lead to a fragmented sense of identity, where the individual feels compelled to adopt multiple personas in order to navigate different social contexts.

Liane Holliday Willey's *Pretending to be Normal* offers a poignant exploration of this internal conflict. Willey's narrative highlights the emotional toll of living a life divided between the authentic self and a carefully constructed mask. For many autistic women, the journey towards self-acceptance involves dismantling these protective layers and allowing their genuine selves to emerge, even in the face of societal judgment.

Empowerment, therefore, becomes a key theme in the discussion of autism in women. Empowerment is not merely about recognition; it is about reclaiming one's narrative and asserting one's right to exist authentically. In recognizing and understanding the female autism phenotype, women can begin to dismantle the internalized stigma and reclaim their identities on their own terms. This process is deeply personal, yet it resonates on a collective level, forging a path toward greater acceptance and inclusivity.

Learning from the Literature: A Tapestry of Voices

The evolution of our understanding of autism in women has been significantly influenced by the voices of those who have experienced it firsthand. In addition to the influential works already mentioned, numerous books and studies have contributed to this growing body of knowledge. For example, the research compiled in *Women and Autism Spectrum Disorder* has shed light on the specific challenges and strengths of autistic women, emphasizing the need for tailored approaches in both clinical practice and everyday life.

Drawing on these diverse sources, we begin to see a richer picture of autism—one that is not confined by outdated stereotypes but is vibrant, complex, and full of potential. The literature reveals that the challenges autistic women face are not merely deficits but are part of a broader narrative of resilience and creativity. This emerging tapestry of voices underscores the importance of listening to and learning from the experiences of autistic women.

Bridging the Gap Between Research and Real Life

The academic and clinical discussions around autism are only one part of the story. The real-world experiences of autistic women— whether shared in memoirs, autobiographies, or personal essays— provide essential context and depth to our understanding. These narratives remind us that behind every diagnosis is a human life filled with dreams, struggles, and triumphs.

For many autistic women, the gap between clinical definitions and lived experience is stark. While research can outline the general characteristics of autism, it is through personal stories that we truly grasp the emotional and social complexities of the condition. Books like *NeuroTribes* and *Pretending to be Normal* have opened the door to these personal narratives, allowing readers to connect with the human side of autism and to see themselves reflected in the stories of others.

As we move forward in our exploration of autism in women, it is crucial to bridge the gap between clinical understanding and personal experience. This integration not only enriches our knowledge but also fosters empathy, understanding, and ultimately, more effective support systems for autistic women.

Conclusion

Defining autism in the context of women requires us to broaden our perspectives, challenge traditional diagnostic models, and embrace the complexity of human neurodiversity. By recognizing the unique characteristics of the female autism phenotype, we pave the way for a more inclusive approach—one that honors both the challenges and the strengths of autistic women.

In this chapter, we have re-examined what autism means, explored how it manifests differently in women, and discussed the societal and diagnostic barriers that have long hindered a full understanding of the condition. We have drawn upon influential texts—from Steve Silberman's *NeuroTribes* to Liane Holliday Willey's *Pretending to be Normal*, and Tony Attwood's *The Complete Guide to Asperger's Syndrome*—to illustrate that the narrative of autism is evolving. This evolution is crucial for developing more sensitive diagnostic tools, better support systems, and a greater appreciation for the diverse ways in which autism can enrich our lives.

As we continue this journey, it is our hope that a deeper understanding of autism in women will empower those who have long felt misunderstood, paving the way for more authentic self-expression and acceptance. In embracing a broader definition of autism, we not only validate the experiences of autistic women but also contribute to a more compassionate and inclusive society—one that values the richness of human diversity in all its forms.

This chapter sets the foundation for the discussions that will follow by challenging conventional definitions and encouraging us to view autism through a more inclusive lens. By engaging with both scientific research and personal narratives, we begin to unravel the intricate tapestry of experiences that define autism in women. The insights gleaned here are vital for anyone seeking to understand or support autistic women—be it as a family member, clinician, or the women themselves—providing a stepping stone towards a future where every voice is heard and every story is valued.

3

Historical Perspectives and Evolving Understandings

Understanding the evolution of autism diagnosis—and particularly its perception in women—requires us to journey through decades of research, cultural norms, and shifting clinical paradigms. This chapter examines the historical context in which autism was studied, the biases that have shaped our current understanding, and the gradual evolution towards a more inclusive perspective that embraces the female autism phenotype.

Early Research and the Male-Centric Paradigm

Autism was first described in the early 20th century by pioneering researchers such as Leo Kanner and Hans Asperger. Kanner's 1943 work painted autism as a rare condition marked by social withdrawal and rigidity, while Asperger's observations, published later, focused on children who exhibited exceptional abilities alongside social challenges. However, both early descriptions predominantly involved boys, reflecting prevailing cultural and scientific biases of the time.

In those early years, the tools and diagnostic criteria developed to identify autism were inherently limited. Researchers, influenced by the norms of mid-20th century society, largely overlooked the possibility that autism might present differently in girls. The assumption was that if a child exhibited certain behaviors, they fit the "autistic mold"—a mold that was primarily constructed based on male behavior. As a result, many girls and women who did not exhibit these overt signs were either misdiagnosed or not diagnosed at all.

Books such as *NeuroTribes: The Legacy of Autism* by Steve Silberman provide an extensive overview of these early misconceptions and highlight how a narrow research focus has contributed to decades of misunderstanding. Silberman's historical account shows that the diagnostic criteria for autism were built around the observable behaviors in boys, leaving little room for the more nuanced expressions often found in females.

The Impact of Stereotypes and Cultural Norms

Cultural stereotypes have long influenced the diagnosis and treatment of autism. Societal expectations about gender roles play a critical role in shaping both behavior and the interpretation of that behavior. For instance, qualities such as shyness, empathy, and a tendency toward introspection are often seen as typical—or even desirable—in girls. As a result, the social struggles that may indicate autism in a boy can be dismissed as "typical girl behavior" in a female.

Liane Holliday Willey's *Pretending to be Normal: Living with Asperger's Syndrome* delves into the personal struggles of masking and camouflaging in order to meet societal expectations. Willey recounts her own experiences of learning to hide her natural behaviors, a theme that resonates with countless women who feel pressured to conform to the gendered norms of emotional expressiveness and sociability. This cultural conditioning has historically contributed to the under-recognition of autism in women, as their coping strategies often mask the signs that clinicians were trained to look for.

Evolution of Diagnostic Criteria

Over the years, the diagnostic criteria for autism have undergone several revisions, each reflecting a deeper understanding of the condition. The publication of the Diagnostic and Statistical Manual of Mental Disorders (DSM) has been a central influence on these changes. Earlier editions of the DSM focused on observable behaviors that were more readily associated with the male presentation of autism. It was only with later editions—and with contributions from researchers who began to recognize the unique experiences of autistic women—that the criteria started to evolve.

One of the turning points in the field was the growing recognition of the "female autism phenotype." This concept, which has been discussed in works like *Women and Autism Spectrum Disorder* by Sarah Hendrickx and colleagues, suggests that autistic women may display a subtler range of symptoms, often internalizing their struggles rather than exhibiting overtly disruptive behaviors. Such insights have prompted clinicians and researchers to revise diagnostic frameworks to better capture the diversity of autistic presentations.

Tony Attwood's *The Complete Guide to Asperger's Syndrome* has been influential in this area as well. Attwood highlights the importance of recognizing that many of the traits associated with Asperger's—and by extension, autism—may manifest differently in women. His work emphasizes the need for diagnostic flexibility and a greater understanding of gender-specific nuances in behavior, further contributing to the gradual reshaping of diagnostic practices.

The Role of Feminist Perspectives in Shaping Understandings

The rise of feminist theory in the latter half of the 20th century brought a critical new lens to the study of psychology and mental health. Feminist scholars began to question the male-centric models that had long dominated scientific research, arguing that women's experiences were being systematically marginalized. This critique extended into the field of autism research, where the lived experiences of autistic women were often dismissed or reinterpreted through a gendered bias.

In this context, works such as *Gendered Perspectives in Autism* (an anthology of essays by various authors) emerged, offering a fresh examination of how gender roles influence the manifestation and interpretation of autism. These perspectives have been crucial in highlighting that the behaviors once deemed "abnormal" in boys may be viewed very differently in girls due to societal expectations. Feminist critiques have also underscored the need to deconstruct stereotypes that pigeonhole women into narrowly defined roles, thereby advocating for a broader, more inclusive understanding of neurodiversity.

Pivotal Moments in Research and Awareness

The latter decades of the 20th century and the early 21st century have witnessed several pivotal moments that have reshaped the understanding of autism in women. Increased advocacy and the rise of neurodiversity movements have challenged traditional narratives and opened up new avenues for research and clinical practice.

For instance, a growing number of autobiographies and memoirs from autistic women have provided firsthand accounts of the challenges they face. These personal narratives have not only enriched the scientific literature but have also served as powerful tools for advocacy. They highlight the discrepancies between clinical expectations and lived reality, urging both clinicians and researchers to adopt a more empathetic and inclusive approach.

Books like *Invisible Women: The Exclusion of Women from Research and the Fight for Change* (while not solely focused on autism) have broadened the conversation about how scientific research has historically sidelined women. This broader critique has encouraged autism researchers to re-examine their methods and assumptions, ultimately leading to more gender-sensitive studies and diagnostic criteria.

Shifting Perspectives: From Deficit to Difference

One of the most significant shifts in understanding autism has been the movement from viewing autistic traits as deficits to recognizing them as differences. This paradigm shift, central to the neurodiversity movement, argues that neurological variations are natural and should be celebrated rather than pathologized. This perspective is especially important when considering the female autism phenotype, which often includes traits that are seen as strengths in other contexts.

Steve Silberman's *NeuroTribes* is a seminal work in this regard, as it challenges the deficit model of autism and promotes a more inclusive, strength-based view of neurodiversity. Silberman's work has resonated with many in the autistic community, particularly women, who have long felt pressured to hide their true selves in order to conform to societal norms. By reframing autism as a natural variation in human neurology, researchers and advocates alike have helped pave the way for more supportive and understanding environments.

Integrating Historical Lessons with Contemporary Practice

The historical journey of autism research offers important lessons for contemporary practice. Recognizing the limitations of past models can guide future research and clinical work, ensuring that the diverse experiences of autistic women are adequately represented and addressed. As historical biases are acknowledged and corrected, there is hope for a more equitable approach to diagnosis, intervention, and support.

Modern diagnostic tools are increasingly incorporating feedback from autistic individuals and their families, many of whom recount experiences of misdiagnosis and misunderstanding. This collaborative approach, which values lived experience as much as clinical observation, is a testament to the progress made over the years. It reflects a broader trend towards participatory research, where the voices of those directly affected by autism play a central role in shaping the future of the field.

In *Pretending to be Normal*, Liane Holliday Willey recounts how her own experiences as an autistic woman were largely invalidated by a medical system that was not equipped to see beyond its preconceptions. Her story—and the stories of countless others—has fueled a call for change, urging researchers and clinicians to adopt more holistic and gender-sensitive practices.

The Role of Policy and Advocacy in Driving Change

Beyond the realms of academic research and clinical practice, policy and advocacy have been instrumental in changing the narrative around autism. Over the past few decades, advocacy groups have worked tirelessly to raise awareness of the unique challenges faced by autistic women, influencing both public policy and funding priorities for autism research.

Legislative efforts in various countries have begun to reflect a more nuanced understanding of autism. These policies are increasingly informed by research that emphasizes the importance of early diagnosis and tailored interventions, particularly for populations that have historically been overlooked. Advocacy organizations have been at the forefront of these changes, using data, personal stories, and public campaigns to push for a more inclusive approach to autism.

Books and research reports that focus on the intersection of gender and autism have played a key role in these advocacy efforts. Their findings have not only informed policy but have also empowered autistic women to advocate for themselves. By shining a light on the historical exclusion of female experiences, these works have helped to foster a more inclusive dialogue about what it means to be autistic.

Looking Forward: A Future of Inclusive Understanding

As we reflect on the historical perspectives of autism, it becomes clear that the journey towards a truly inclusive understanding is ongoing. The biases and limitations of past research have left their mark, but they have also provided a roadmap for future progress. Today's researchers, clinicians, and advocates are building on the lessons of history to create diagnostic criteria and support systems that recognize and honor the full spectrum of autistic experiences.

The work of contemporary authors and researchers, including those highlighted in *Women and Autism Spectrum Disorder* and other emerging studies, points to a future where autistic women are no longer relegated to the margins. Instead, their experiences and strengths are being recognized as integral to our understanding of human diversity. This evolving narrative is a testament to the power of advocacy, research, and the courage of individuals who have shared their stories despite decades of silence.

Conclusion

The historical perspectives and evolving understandings of autism in women offer a compelling narrative of both struggle and progress. From the early days of male-centric research to the modern embrace of neurodiversity and strength-based perspectives, the journey has been long and often fraught with challenges. Yet, each step forward represents a victory for those who have been overlooked and misunderstood for far too long.

By reflecting on the historical context and acknowledging the biases that have shaped our current understanding, we are better equipped to forge a future that is both inclusive and empowering. The evolution of diagnostic criteria, the integration of feminist perspectives, and the relentless advocacy efforts all converge to create a richer, more nuanced picture of autism—one that honors the unique experiences of autistic women.

In revisiting seminal works like *NeuroTribes*, *Pretending to be Normal*, and *The Complete Guide to Asperger's Syndrome*, we are reminded that the narrative of autism is not static. It is a dynamic tapestry woven from decades of research, personal struggle, and collective advocacy. As we look to the future, the lessons of the past serve not only as a reminder of what has been lost but also as a beacon guiding us toward a more equitable and compassionate understanding of neurodiversity.

Ultimately, the historical journey is a call to action. It challenges us to question established norms, to listen deeply to the voices of those who have been silenced, and to embrace the complexity and beauty inherent in the human mind. With each new study, each personal narrative, and each policy change, we move closer to a world where every autistic individual—especially women—can thrive, free from the constraints of outdated stereotypes and narrow diagnostic criteria.

The history of autism is a story of transformation, and the future promises even greater strides toward understanding and acceptance. As we continue to build on this legacy, we invite you to join us in exploring the rich, multifaceted narrative of autism in women—a narrative that is as inspiring as it is necessary.

This chapter has traced the historical evolution of autism research, revealing how initial biases and narrow diagnostic criteria contributed to the under-recognition of autistic women. By examining the interplay between cultural norms, early research, and evolving diagnostic practices, we gain crucial insights into the forces that have shaped—and are continuing to reshape—the understanding of the female autism phenotype. With a foundation built on both academic research and personal narratives, this exploration sets the stage for a future where every voice is heard, every difference is valued, and every individual has the opportunity to flourish.

4

The Art of Masking – Camouflaging Autism

For many autistic women, the act of masking—consciously or unconsciously concealing traits that diverge from societal norms—has long been a survival strategy. This chapter delves into the intricate art of masking: what it is, why it is so pervasive among autistic women, and how it affects their mental, emotional, and social lives. We will examine the layers of camouflaging behavior, discuss its historical and cultural roots, and consider both its short-term benefits and long-term consequences. In doing so, we draw upon personal narratives and influential texts, including Liane Holliday Willey's Pretending to be Normal: Living with Asperger's Syndrome, Tony Attwood's insights in The Complete Guide to Asperger's Syndrome, and Steve Silberman's NeuroTribes: The Legacy of Autism, among others.

Understanding Masking: A Protective Mechanism

Masking refers to the practice of hiding or compensating for one's natural behaviors and traits in order to blend into social settings. For autistic women, this might involve mimicking neurotypical expressions, rehearsing social interactions, or suppressing sensory reactions that might be deemed "unusual." At its core, masking is a protective mechanism—a way to navigate a world that often values conformity over authenticity.

Liane Holliday Willey's memoir, *Pretending to be Normal*, vividly illustrates the toll that masking can take on one's identity. Willey recounts the painstaking effort required to emulate social behaviors that never come naturally, highlighting how masking can create a chasm between one's inner self and external presentation. This separation, while useful in evading immediate social rejection, can lead to a profound sense of disconnection and emotional exhaustion over time.

Why Masking Occurs

Societal Expectations and Gender Norms

One of the primary drivers of masking in autistic women is societal pressure. From a young age, girls are often socialized to be accommodating, empathetic, and compliant. These expectations compel many autistic girls and women to hide behaviors that deviate from these norms. For instance, while a lack of eye contact or a reserved demeanor might be flagged as a red flag in boys, these traits can be misinterpreted as shyness or politeness in girls. In striving to conform to these gendered expectations, many autistic women learn to adopt a facade that conceals their true selves.

In *NeuroTribes*, Steve Silberman discusses how early research into autism was overwhelmingly based on observations of boys, creating diagnostic criteria that failed to capture the nuances of female presentation. This gap has meant that autistic women have had to develop masking techniques as a way to avoid misdiagnosis or being labeled as "abnormal."

The Need for Social Acceptance

Humans are inherently social creatures, and the drive for acceptance is powerful. For autistic women, the risk of social isolation is heightened by the fear of being misunderstood or rejected. Masking becomes a tool to gain social approval, to navigate school, work, and personal relationships without drawing unwanted attention to behaviors that might be deemed nonconforming. Tony Attwood, in *The Complete Guide to Asperger's Syndrome*, explains that many autistic individuals— especially women—use masking as a way to secure their place in social hierarchies. However, this constant performance can lead to significant psychological strain.

Coping with Sensory Overload

Beyond social acceptance, many autistic women mask to manage sensory overload. In environments where the noise, lights, or even the pace of conversation can be overwhelming, masking offers a way to minimize visible reactions. For instance, suppressing a startle response to sudden loud sounds or forcing a neutral expression when experiencing sensory distress can help maintain a semblance of normalcy in public spaces. Although these strategies can be effective in the short term, they often require tremendous mental energy, leading to fatigue and burnout.

The Many Faces of Masking

Behavioral Camouflage

Behavioral camouflage is perhaps the most visible form of masking. This includes imitating body language, facial expressions, and speech patterns of neurotypical peers. Many autistic women spend years—or even decades—practicing these behaviors until they become second nature. The challenge, however, lies in the constant need to adapt and modify one's behavior depending on the social context. In doing so, authentic expressions of emotion and personality may become suppressed.

For example, an autistic woman might learn to smile in social situations even when she feels anxious or overwhelmed. Over time, this habitual smiling can mask underlying distress, making it difficult for both herself and others to recognize when she is struggling. As Willey describes in *Pretending to be Normal*, the pressure to maintain this facade can be relentless, often leading to internal turmoil and a diminished sense of self.

Verbal and Nonverbal Mimicry

Another aspect of masking involves mimicking both verbal and nonverbal communication. This might mean rehearsing conversational scripts or deliberately imitating the intonation and rhythm of speech that is considered "normal." Nonverbal mimicry, such as adopting expected facial expressions or gesturing in socially acceptable ways, is equally important. Although these strategies can facilitate smoother social interactions, they also contribute to the internal conflict many autistic women feel—between who they truly are and who they feel pressured to be.

Suppression of Stimming

Stimming—repetitive behaviors or movements that help regulate sensory input and emotion—is a common trait among autistic individuals. For many autistic women, stimming behaviors like hand-flapping, rocking, or fidgeting are sources of comfort and self-regulation. However, societal disapproval often forces them to hide these behaviors. The suppression of stimming is a prime example of how masking extends beyond social interactions; it infiltrates personal coping mechanisms that are vital for emotional balance. The constant suppression can lead to increased stress and a reduction in overall well-being, as natural self-soothing methods are stifled.

The Long-Term Consequences of Masking

While masking can provide immediate benefits—such as improved social acceptance or reduced conflict—it often comes at a steep price over the long term. The ongoing effort to appear "normal" can lead to chronic anxiety, depression, and even identity confusion. Many autistic women report feeling as though they are living two lives: one for the public and one that remains hidden from the world. This duality creates a persistent internal tension, where the energy required to maintain the mask leaves little reserve for authentic self-expression.

Moreover, prolonged masking can delay or complicate the process of receiving an accurate diagnosis. When clinicians rely on observable behaviors, the subtleties hidden behind a mask can result in misdiagnosis or complete oversight of autism. This diagnostic delay not only hampers access to tailored support and interventions but also reinforces the individual's belief that something is inherently wrong with them. Tony Attwood discusses this phenomenon in *The Complete Guide to Asperger's Syndrome*, noting that the very skills developed to cope with social expectations can obscure the underlying neurodiversity.

Personal Narratives: The Hidden Toll of Masking

The stories of countless autistic women underscore the deep personal toll that masking can take. Many recount a childhood spent meticulously observing and imitating peers, a constant effort to fit in, and an eventual realization that this constant performance had come at the cost of their authenticity. One woman described her experience as "always acting, never being," a sentiment echoed in numerous personal essays and memoirs. These narratives illustrate how masking is not merely a set of behaviors, but a profound, ongoing struggle with identity.

For example, consider the story of Clara (a pseudonym), who spent years perfecting her social script. Despite excelling in academic and professional settings, she constantly battled an inner sense of isolation and exhaustion. Clara's experience is a stark reminder that masking, while outwardly successful, often masks a profound inner distress. Her story, like those found in autobiographical works and support group discussions, is a powerful testament to the resilience—and the vulnerability—of autistic women.

Strategies for Unmasking and Self-Acceptance

Given the high cost of masking, many autistic women eventually seek ways to unmask and embrace their authentic selves. The journey toward unmasking is complex and deeply personal, often involving therapy, peer support, and self-reflection. Several strategies can help facilitate this process:

Therapeutic Approaches

Therapies such as cognitive behavioral therapy (CBT) and acceptance and commitment therapy (ACT) can provide tools to manage the anxiety associated with unmasking. These approaches encourage individuals to accept their neurodivergence and develop strategies for expressing their true selves in a safe environment. Clinical work described in *The Complete Guide to Asperger's Syndrome* highlights the importance of tailoring therapy to address the unique challenges of masking and the need for a compassionate, individualized approach.

Peer Support and Community

Connecting with others who share similar experiences can be trans-formative. Peer support groups—both online and in person—offer safe spaces for autistic women to share their struggles and triumphs without fear of judgment. The neurodiversity movement, as detailed in *NeuroTribes*, has fostered a community where differences are celebrated rather than hidden. Hearing others' stories of unmasking can provide the courage and inspiration needed to take similar steps toward authenticity.

Building Self-Awareness

Self-awareness is a critical step toward unmasking. Journaling, mindful-ness, and reflective practices can help individuals identify the moments when they are masking and explore the underlying reasons. Understand-ing these triggers is essential for developing healthier coping strategies. By recognizing the signs of masking, autistic women can gradually learn to lower the mask and let their genuine selves emerge.

Redefining Success and Normalcy

A key component of unmasking involves redefining what it means to be "normal" or "successful." Instead of striving to meet neurotypical standards, many autistic women are finding empowerment in celebrating their unique strengths and perspectives. This redefinition is at the heart of the neurodiversity movement. Works like *NeuroTribes* encourage us to see autism not as a deficiency, but as a different—and equally valuable—way of experiencing the world.

The Duality of Masking: Benefits and Costs

It is important to acknowledge that masking, for all its costs, also serves as an adaptive mechanism. In many situations, it can protect autistic women from bullying, discrimination, or misunderstanding. For instance, in professional environments where conformity is rewarded, masking might open doors that would otherwise remain closed. However, these short-term gains must be weighed against the long-term costs. The emotional labor required to maintain a mask can lead to burnout and a diminished sense of self-worth.

Many authors and clinicians emphasize that the goal is not necessarily to eliminate masking entirely but to achieve a balance. By learning when and where it is safe or necessary to mask—and when it is healthier to be authentic—autistic women can better manage the social demands of daily life. This balance allows for self-advocacy and the pursuit of personal goals without the constant burden of hiding one's true identity.

Looking Toward a More Inclusive Future

The discussion around masking is part of a larger conversation about acceptance, diversity, and the need for societal change. As awareness grows about the unique challenges faced by autistic women, there is an increasing call for environments that allow for authenticity. Schools, workplaces, and social institutions are gradually recognizing the value of neurodiversity and adapting their practices accordingly.

Educational reforms, for instance, are beginning to incorporate individualized learning strategies that respect the sensory and social needs of autistic students. Similarly, workplace policies are evolving to include flexible environments and support systems that enable autistic employees to thrive without the constant pressure to mask. The collective efforts of advocates, researchers, and community leaders are paving the way for a future where the art of masking becomes less necessary because authenticity is valued.

Conclusion

The art of masking is a multifaceted and deeply personal strategy that has allowed many autistic women to navigate a world that often misunderstands them. While masking can open doors to social acceptance and professional success, it comes with a significant emotional toll. The constant effort to hide one's true self can lead to chronic stress, identity confusion, and mental health challenges—a cost that many autistic women pay silently for years.

Drawing on insights from *Pretending to be Normal*, *NeuroTribes*, and *The Complete Guide to Asperger's Syndrome*, this chapter has explored the reasons behind masking, its various manifestations, and the profound impact it has on the lives of autistic women. It has also highlighted the potential for unmasking through therapy, community support, and a redefinition of what it means to be "normal." By understanding both the adaptive benefits and the personal costs of masking, we can move toward a more compassionate and inclusive approach—one that celebrates authenticity and recognizes the rich diversity of human experience.

As we continue our journey through the female autism spectrum, it is our hope that this exploration of masking serves as both a validation of individual experiences and a call to action. A call to create environments where the need for masking is diminished, where autistic women can express themselves freely, and where the unique strengths that come with neurodiversity are embraced. The path toward unmasking is not about rejecting social norms altogether, but rather about reclaiming one's narrative and redefining success on one's own terms.

In embracing this journey, we honor the courage of every autistic woman who has struggled in silence and emerges each day with resilience. Their stories are a powerful reminder that the quest for authenticity is both deeply personal and universally significant—a quest that enriches our collective understanding of what it means to be human.

This chapter has delved into the complexities of masking, illustrating how autistic women navigate a delicate balance between societal expectations and personal authenticity. By drawing on influential works and personal narratives, we have unpacked the many layers of camouflaging behavior, its origins, and its long-lasting impacts. As the conversation around autism continues to evolve, it is essential to remember that the art of masking is not a flaw, but a survival strategy—a testament to the strength and resilience of those who must, day after day, perform for a world that has yet to fully understand them.

5

Unveiling the Female Autism Phenotype

The female autism phenotype has emerged as a vital concept in understanding the full spectrum of autism. In this chapter, we explore the unique ways autism manifests in women and girls—ways that are often subtle, internalized, and easily overlooked. By examining clinical insights, personal narratives, and scholarly work, we aim to illuminate the distinctive characteristics of the female autism phenotype, celebrate the strengths that come with neurodiversity, and address the challenges that have long contributed to misdiagnosis and misunderstanding.

A Different Manifestation of Autism

Traditionally, autism has been defined by characteristics such as overt social difficulties, repetitive behaviors, and distinct communication challenges. However, as researchers and clinicians have expanded their understanding of the condition, it has become clear that the expression of autism in women can differ markedly from that observed in men. Rather than fitting neatly into the conventional diagnostic mold, many autistic women display traits that are more nuanced and often internalized.

For example, whereas a male on the spectrum might exhibit clear repetitive motions or insistence on sameness, an autistic woman may engage in subtler forms of repetitive behavior—such as an intense focus on a hobby or an unusual fixation on details—that can easily be mistaken for passion or meticulousness. As Liane Holliday Willey explains in *Pretending to be Normal: Living with Asperger's Syndrome*, many autistic women have learned to mask their difficulties by developing advanced social skills and adaptive strategies that, while impressive, often conceal the underlying neurodivergence.

Internal Experiences vs. External Presentation

One of the most striking aspects of the female autism phenotype is the gap between internal experience and external presentation. Many autistic women report a rich inner life filled with intense sensory perceptions, deep emotional currents, and vivid imagination. Yet outwardly, they may appear to conform to social norms—smiling in social situations, engaging in conversations, and even excelling in academic or professional settings.

This dissonance is a core challenge. The internal world of an autistic woman can be tumultuous and overwhelming, filled with sensory overload, anxiety, and the constant pressure to appear "normal." Meanwhile, her external behavior—honed through years of practice and masking—may hide these struggles from friends, family, and clinicians. In *NeuroTribes: The Legacy of Autism*, Steve Silberman emphasizes that the traditional understanding of autism has been skewed by the emphasis on observable behaviors. For autistic women, who often camouflage their true selves, the external calm can belie internal chaos.

The Role of Social Conditioning

Social expectations play a significant role in shaping the female autism phenotype. From early childhood, girls are socialized to be nurturing, communicative, and socially adept. These cultural pressures compel many autistic girls to adopt behaviors that, while facilitating acceptance, also hide their natural neurological differences. This phenomenon is not a deliberate choice but rather a survival strategy—a way to avoid stigma and the isolation that often accompanies deviation from social norms.

Books like *Women and Autism Spectrum Disorder* by Sarah Hendrickx and colleagues illustrate how these societal expectations force autistic girls and women to perform a version of normalcy. They learn early on that their natural tendencies—such as a preference for solitude or deep focus on niche interests—might lead to criticism or misunderstanding if expressed openly. Over time, the constant effort to fit into a neurotypical mold leads to the development of a distinctly female presentation of autism—one that is both adaptive and, unfortunately, often under-recognized.

Unique Characteristics of the Female Autism Phenotype

Several key features help define the female autism phenotype:

Subtle Social Difficulties

Autistic women frequently experience social challenges that are less visible than those traditionally associated with autism. They might have difficulty initiating conversations, interpreting subtle social cues, or maintaining friendships, yet these issues often go unnoticed because they are masked by learned social skills. Their challenges are not in the lack of desire to connect but in the complexity of navigating social nuances. This subtlety can result in chronic feelings of isolation and misunderstanding, as the very behaviors that signal distress are hidden behind a veneer of competence.

Exceptional Empathy and Sensitivity

Paradoxically, many autistic women are noted for their deep empathy and sensitivity. While empathy is often seen as a strength, in the context of autism it can also lead to emotional overwhelm. The ability to absorb the emotions of others, combined with personal sensory sensitivities, can create a heightened state of stress and anxiety. In Tony Attwood's *The Complete Guide to Asperger's Syndrome*, the interplay between empathy and sensory overload is highlighted as a double-edged sword—contributing both to rich interpersonal insights and significant emotional fatigue.

Intense and Focused Interests

Another hallmark of the female autism phenotype is the presence of intense, focused interests. These interests often align with culturally accepted pursuits—such as literature, art, or animals—making them appear less atypical. However, beneath the surface, these interests can be all-consuming and serve as a critical coping mechanism. They provide structure, comfort, and a way to engage with the world that is deeply personal. This intensity, while sometimes misunderstood by those unfamiliar with autism, is a powerful testament to the unique cognitive strengths of autistic women.

Advanced Coping and Masking Strategies

As discussed in previous chapters, masking is a central feature of the female autism phenotype. Autistic women often develop highly sophisticated methods of compensating for social difficulties. These strategies include mimicking body language, rehearsing conversations, and even suppressing stimming behaviors. While these adaptive techniques can facilitate social interaction, they also contribute to a disconnect between the inner and outer self. Over time, the energy expended on masking can lead to emotional burnout and a fractured sense of identity.

The Impact of Misdiagnosis

One of the most troubling aspects of the female autism phenotype is its role in delayed or missed diagnoses. Because many of the signs are subtle or masked, autistic women are frequently misdiagnosed with other conditions such as anxiety, depression, or borderline personality disorder. These misdiagnoses not only delay access to appropriate support but also reinforce feelings of inadequacy and self-doubt.

The narratives collected in *Pretending to be Normal* and other autobiographical accounts highlight a recurring theme: the struggle for validation. Autistic women often spend years, sometimes decades, questioning their own experiences because the external behaviors that should trigger a diagnosis are hidden behind a learned façade. This diagnostic oversight is a stark reminder of the need for clinicians to consider the unique presentation of autism in women—a call that is echoed in emerging research and advocacy efforts.

Celebrating Neurodiversity

While the challenges associated with the female autism phenotype are significant, it is equally important to celebrate the unique strengths that accompany these differences. The intense focus, empathy, and creative thinking often seen in autistic women can be tremendous assets in both personal and professional realms. The neurodiversity movement, as explored in *NeuroTribes*, encourages us to view these traits not as deficits but as variations that enrich our collective human experience.

Embracing neurodiversity means recognizing that there is no single "correct" way to be human. Autistic women, with their unique cognitive styles and sensory perceptions, contribute perspectives that are invaluable in a rapidly changing world. Their ability to think differently can lead to innovation and creative problem-solving, challenging conventional wisdom and opening new avenues for understanding and progress.

Personal Narratives and Real-World Implications

The lived experiences of autistic women provide powerful insights into the female autism phenotype. Consider the story of Emma (a pseudonym), who describes feeling "invisible" in social settings despite her vibrant inner life. Emma's account, echoed in various memoirs and personal essays, underscores the loneliness and isolation that can result from years of masking. Yet, her story also reveals moments of profound clarity—when, in safe and accepting environments, she is able to let go of the mask and connect authentically with others.

These personal narratives are critical in shifting the conversation about autism. They challenge the narrow definitions that have long dominated clinical practice and call for a more inclusive approach that honors the full spectrum of human experience. In *Women and*

Autism Spectrum Disorder, the authors compile stories from women who have navigated the challenges of a misaligned diagnostic framework, advocating for a model that truly reflects the diversity of the autistic experience.

Bridging Research and Practice

A major challenge moving forward is ensuring that the insights gained from research on the female autism phenotype translate into better clinical practices and social support systems. Current diagnostic tools are increasingly being re-evaluated in light of new findings, and clinicians are gradually being trained to recognize the subtleties of autism in women. However, there remains a significant gap between research and real-world application.

In *The Complete Guide to Asperger's Syndrome*, Tony Attwood emphasizes the need for ongoing education and awareness among healthcare professionals. By integrating the latest research with clinical training, it is possible to develop diagnostic frameworks that are sensitive to gender differences. This evolution in practice is not just a matter of scientific accuracy—it is a matter of social justice, ensuring that autistic women receive the recognition and support they deserve.

Toward a More Inclusive Future

Unveiling the female autism phenotype is a crucial step in creating a society that values and supports all forms of neurodiversity. As we continue to refine our understanding of autism, it is essential that we challenge outdated assumptions and embrace a more nuanced view of what it means to be autistic. This shift requires collaboration between researchers, clinicians, educators, and, most importantly, autistic women themselves.

The road ahead involves not only refining diagnostic criteria but also creating environments where autistic women can thrive. Educational institutions, workplaces, and social systems must adapt to accommodate different cognitive styles and sensory needs. Advocacy efforts and public awareness campaigns play a vital role in driving this change, helping to dismantle the stereotypes that have long marginalized autistic women.

The female autism phenotype is a multifaceted and dynamic concept that challenges the traditional understanding of autism. By acknowledging the unique ways in which autism manifests in women—through subtle social difficulties, intense internal experiences, and advanced masking strategies—we begin to see the full spectrum of neurodiversity. Influential works such as *Pretending to be Normal*, *NeuroTribes*, and *The Complete Guide to Asperger's Syndrome* have all contributed to this evolving narrative, offering insights that empower autistic women and advocate for a more inclusive diagnostic framework.

In celebrating the unique strengths of the female autism phenotype—empathy, creativity, and deep passion—we also confront the challenges of misdiagnosis and the emotional toll of masking. Personal narratives, woven through clinical research and memoir, remind us that every autistic woman has a story worth hearing. As we move forward, bridging the gap between research and practice is paramount. Only by integrating these insights into everyday life can we create a world where the diversity of human experience is not just acknowledged, but embraced.

In redefining autism to include the nuances of the female experience, we honor the resilience and brilliance of autistic women everywhere. Their journeys, fraught with challenges yet marked by extraordinary strength, inspire us to rethink what it means to be different—and to value difference as an essential part of our shared humanity.

By unveiling the female autism phenotype, we take a crucial step toward a future where every autistic individual is seen, supported, and celebrated for who they truly are.

6

The Diagnostic Journey – Challenges and Breakthroughs

The diagnostic journey for autistic women is often long, convoluted, and laden with obstacles. In this chapter, we explore the intricacies of arriving at a diagnosis—from the limitations of traditional diagnostic criteria to the personal and systemic challenges that many autistic women face. We delve into how misdiagnosis, delayed recognition, and evolving diagnostic frameworks shape the lives of those on the female spectrum. Drawing on insights from influential works such as Pretending to be Normal: Living with Asperger's Syndrome by Liane Holliday Willey, The Complete Guide to Asperger's Syndrome by Tony Attwood, and NeuroTribes: The Legacy of Autism by Steve Silberman, we illuminate both the struggles and the breakthroughs in understanding autism in women.

The Early Struggle: Seeking Recognition in a Male-Centric System

For decades, autism research and clinical practice were dominated by a male-centric model of the condition. Early diagnostic criteria—developed primarily through studies of boys—placed emphasis on overt behaviors such as repetitive movements, social withdrawal, and language delays. These criteria, while effective for many, have consistently overlooked the subtler presentation seen in many autistic women. In *NeuroTribes*, Steve Silberman illustrates how historical biases led to diagnostic models that could miss or misinterpret the nuanced behaviors of girls, resulting in many women being left without answers for years.

Many autistic women recount their childhoods as periods of internal struggle masked by external conformity. They often experienced significant social and sensory challenges without receiving the validation that comes with a diagnosis. Instead, they were labeled as "shy," "anxious," or even "eccentric." This lack of recognition is poignantly described in Liane Holliday Willey's *Pretending to be Normal*, where she details her personal odyssey of years spent adapting and camouflaging her behaviors just to fit in—a survival mechanism that, while effective in the short term, often led to deep-seated self-doubt.

The Diagnostic Criteria: Limitations and Evolving Understanding

Traditional diagnostic tools, such as the criteria outlined in the Diagnostic and Statistical Manual of Mental Disorders (DSM), have long been critiqued for their inability to capture the full range of autistic presentations. These tools were built around observable, often overt behaviors that are more common in boys, such as repetitive actions or significant language delays. In contrast, many autistic women present with less conspicuous signs—developing coping strategies that mask their struggles, engaging in interests that appear socially acceptable, or internalizing their difficulties until emotional distress peaks.

Tony Attwood's *The Complete Guide to Asperger's Syndrome* has been influential in highlighting how these diagnostic criteria can miss critical subtleties. Attwood emphasizes that while the core challenges of autism remain consistent, the way they manifest in women can be deeply influenced by societal expectations and personal coping mechanisms. This disconnect between internal experience and external behavior often results in women being misdiagnosed with anxiety, depression, or borderline personality disorder, rather than receiving the correct autism diagnosis.

The Journey to Diagnosis: Personal Narratives and Systemic Barriers

The path to an accurate diagnosis for many autistic women is often marked by repeated missteps. Personal narratives, such as those shared in *Pretending to be Normal*, reveal a recurring pattern: years of feeling misunderstood, invalidated, and forced to "pretend" in order to navigate a neurotypical world. These stories are a testament to the resilience of autistic women, but they also highlight the cost of delayed diagnosis. The longer an individual goes without recognition, the more likely it is that they develop secondary mental health challenges—such as anxiety, depression, or chronic burnout—stemming from years of masking and internalizing stress.

One common thread in these narratives is the experience of "diagnostic overshadowing," where symptoms of autism are overshadowed by, or attributed solely to, other conditions. For instance, a young woman might be treated for anxiety without clinicians ever exploring the possibility of autism. This phenomenon not only delays appropriate support but also compounds the individual's sense of isolation and frustration.

Moreover, the diagnostic process itself can be disempowering. Many autistic women report feeling as though they must "earn" their diagnosis by conforming to criteria that do not fully capture their experiences. They are often required to "prove" their differences in clinical settings that are not designed to reveal the complexities of their inner worlds. This gap between clinical observation and lived reality leaves many feeling invisible and misunderstood—a sentiment echoed throughout both memoirs and clinical case studies.

Systemic Challenges: Biases and the Need for Change

Beyond the limitations of diagnostic criteria lie systemic challenges that continue to hinder accurate and timely diagnoses. The healthcare system, with its long-standing emphasis on male presentations of autism, frequently lacks the training and awareness needed to identify the female autism phenotype. As discussed in *Women and Autism Spectrum Disorder* by Sarah Hendrickx and colleagues, there is a pressing need for clinicians to adopt gender-sensitive diagnostic approaches that account for the unique manifestations of autism in women.

A critical component of this systemic issue is the lack of representation in research. Historically, studies on autism have underrepresented females, leading to a skewed understanding of the condition. This research gap reinforces the diagnostic bias and leaves clinicians without the robust, evidence-based guidelines needed to recognize autism in women. The ongoing efforts to bridge this gap are beginning to show promise, but the transformation is gradual. Researchers and clinicians are increasingly advocating for more inclusive studies and the development of diagnostic tools that reflect the diversity of the autistic experience.

Breakthroughs in Diagnosis: A New Era of Understanding

Despite these challenges, there has been significant progress in recent years. As awareness of the female autism phenotype grows, so too does the development of more nuanced diagnostic tools and practices. Clinicians are becoming more adept at recognizing the subtleties of autism in women—whether through revised clinical guidelines, improved screening methods, or the integration of self-reported experiences into diagnostic evaluations.

The shift toward neurodiversity—a concept eloquently championed in *NeuroTribes*—has also been pivotal in transforming the diagnostic landscape. Neurodiversity posits that neurological differences, including autism, should be viewed as natural variations rather than disorders to be "fixed." This perspective not only challenges the deficit-based models of the past but also empowers autistic individuals to embrace their unique strengths and advocate for themselves. For many autistic women, receiving a diagnosis later in life, though frustrating, becomes a turning point—a moment of clarity that validates years of internal struggle and offers a path toward self-acceptance and tailored support.

Modern diagnostic approaches increasingly incorporate a multi-dimensional view of autism. Rather than relying solely on observable behaviors, clinicians are now considering the individual's internal experiences, sensory sensitivities, and the impact of masking. This holistic approach is more likely to capture the full spectrum of autistic experiences, particularly in women whose symptoms may not align with traditional expectations. As Tony Attwood notes in *The Complete Guide to Asperger's Syndrome*, this evolution in diagnostic practice is essential for providing the right support at the right time.

The Role of Self-Advocacy and Peer Support

One of the most transformative aspects of the diagnostic journey for many autistic women is the role of self-advocacy. With the rise of online communities, social media, and peer support groups, countless women have found solidarity and validation in shared experiences. These platforms offer safe spaces to discuss symptoms, exchange coping strategies, and ultimately challenge the stigma surrounding autism.

Personal accounts shared in online forums and support groups often detail the empowerment that comes with finally receiving a diagnosis. For many, this milestone is not just a label—it is a gateway to understanding their own needs, seeking appropriate accommodations, and finding communities that embrace neurodiversity. The stories of these women, as documented in various autobiographies and online memoirs, serve as powerful reminders of the importance of self-advocacy in the face of systemic shortcomings.

The collective movement toward greater awareness and understanding has also spurred efforts to educate clinicians and policymakers. Advocacy groups and research institutions are increasingly emphasizing the need for gender-sensitive training in medical schools and continuing education for practicing clinicians. These initiatives are critical for transforming the diagnostic process from one that is exclusionary and narrow to one that is inclusive and representative of all autistic experiences.

Navigating the Diagnostic Process: Practical Considerations

For those embarking on the diagnostic journey, the process can be both daunting and liberating. It often involves multiple evaluations, consultations with various specialists, and a considerable amount of self-reflection. Here are some practical strategies and considerations for navigating this complex landscape:

- **Documenting Personal Experiences:**
- Keeping a detailed journal of your experiences—covering sensory sensitivities, social challenges, and emotional responses—can be invaluable. These records provide concrete examples for clinicians and help ensure that the subtleties of your experiences are not overlooked.
- **Seeking Clinicians with Expertise in Female Autism:**
- Look for healthcare professionals who have a track record of working with autistic women. Their familiarity with the female autism phenotype can lead to a more accurate and empathetic assessment.
- **Advocating for Comprehensive Evaluations:**
- Don't hesitate to ask for a multi-disciplinary evaluation that considers both psychological and sensory aspects. A comprehensive approach can help uncover the hidden layers of autism that standard assessments might miss.
- **Connecting with Support Networks:**
- Joining support groups—whether online or in person—can provide emotional support and practical advice during the diagnostic process. Hearing the stories of others who have navigated similar challenges can offer both comfort and guidance.
- **Educating Oneself About Autism:**
- Familiarize yourself with key texts like *Pretending to be Normal*, *The Complete Guide to Asperger's Syndrome*, and *NeuroTribes*. These works not only provide insight into the condition but also serve as tools for self-advocacy and empowerment.

The Promise of a Better Future

The challenges faced in diagnosing autism in women underscore a broader need for systemic change. As our understanding of neuro-diversity deepens, so too does the promise of a future where every autistic individual is recognized for who they are. The breakthroughs in diagnostic practices, fueled by both clinical innovation and grassroots advocacy, represent a shift toward a more inclusive and compassionate healthcare system.

This new era is characterized by a collaborative approach—one that values the insights of autistic individuals themselves. By listening to personal narratives and integrating them into clinical practice, the medical community is moving closer to a model of diagnosis that is as diverse as the people it seeks to serve. This paradigm shift is not just about improving diagnostic accuracy; it is about ensuring that every person receives the understanding, respect, and support they deserve.

Reflections on the Journey

The diagnostic journey is deeply personal, yet it is also a reflection of broader societal and systemic issues. For many autistic women, the path to a correct diagnosis is filled with frustration, self-doubt, and the burden of masking. But it is also a journey of self-discovery—a process of peeling back layers of misunderstanding to reveal an authentic self that has long been obscured by societal expectations.

The narratives that emerge from this journey are powerful. They speak of resilience in the face of adversity, of the courage to demand recognition, and of the transformative impact that a correct diagnosis can have. These stories remind us that while the road may be long and fraught with obstacles, each step forward is a victory—not just for the individual, but for the entire community advocating for neurodiversity.

Concluding thoughts

The diagnostic journey for autistic women is emblematic of the challenges inherent in recognizing and validating diverse human experiences. As we have seen throughout this chapter, the path to diagnosis is marked by systemic biases, outdated diagnostic criteria, and the personal toll of masking. Yet, amidst these challenges, there is a growing movement toward understanding and inclusion—one that draws on both groundbreaking research and the lived experiences of those on the spectrum.

Influential works such as *Pretending to be Normal*, *The Complete Guide to Asperger's Syndrome*, and *NeuroTribes* have been instrumental in shifting the conversation and paving the way for a more accurate, empathetic, and inclusive approach to diagnosis. The progress made so far offers hope for a future where every autistic individual, regardless of gender, can receive the support and recognition they need from the very beginning of their journey.

Ultimately, the diagnostic journey is not merely a clinical process—it is a transformative experience that empowers autistic women to reclaim their narratives and advocate for their rightful place in society. With continued advocacy, education, and systemic reform, we move closer to a world where the unique strengths of the female autism phenotype are not only recognized but celebrated.

In embracing the challenges and breakthroughs of the diagnostic journey, we honor the resilience of those who have long fought to be seen and understood. Their stories serve as a call to action—a reminder that true progress lies in creating a society where diversity in all its forms is acknowledged, valued, and nurtured.

This chapter has navigated the complex landscape of autism diagnosis for women, shedding light on the historical biases, systemic challenges, and transformative breakthroughs that shape the journey. By integrating personal narratives with clinical insights and drawing on seminal works in the field, we have explored the multifaceted process of arriving at an accurate diagnosis. As we continue to refine our understanding and practices, the hope is that future generations of autistic women will no longer face the same hurdles, but will instead find a path to recognition and support that is as unique and diverse as they are.

7

Relationships and Social Navigation

Relationships are a cornerstone of human experience, yet for autistic women, navigating the intricate web of social connections can be particularly challenging. In this chapter, we explore the nuances of family dynamics, friendships, romantic relationships, and everyday communication for autistic women. We delve into how masking, societal expectations, and the unique traits of the female autism phenotype influence these interactions. Drawing on personal narratives and influential works—such as Liane Holliday Willey's Pretending to be Normal: Living with Asperger's Syndrome, Tony Attwood's The Complete Guide to Asperger's Syndrome, and Steve Silberman's NeuroTribes: The Legacy of Autism—we examine both the obstacles and the opportunities that arise when forging connections in a neurotypical world.

The Foundation of Relationships: Family Dynamics

Family is often the first arena in which autistic women learn to interact with the world. For many, the family environment is a double-edged sword. On one hand, it can be a source of unconditional love and acceptance; on the other, it can magnify the pressures to conform to social norms. Many autistic women recount childhood experiences where their behaviors were misinterpreted as stubbornness or emotional instability, rather than recognized as manifestations of their neurodivergence.

In *Pretending to be Normal*, Liane Holliday Willey describes the constant balancing act of trying to meet parental and societal expectations while grappling with internal sensory and emotional challenges. This dynamic often leads to a situation where the autistic daughter feels compelled to "perform" normalcy—suppressing natural behaviors in order to avoid conflict or disappointment. Parents, often unaware of the subtle signs of autism in girls, may inadvertently reinforce these behaviors, leaving their daughters feeling isolated and misunderstood.

Despite these challenges, family relationships also offer a foundation for growth and acceptance. When parents, siblings, and extended family members make the effort to understand the unique needs of an autistic daughter, they create an environment in which she can explore her identity with greater authenticity. Increasingly, resources and support groups—like those discussed in *Women and Autism Spectrum Disorder*—are guiding families on how to nurture and celebrate neurodiversity within the home.

Friendships: The Delicate Dance of Connection

Friendships are central to social well-being, yet they can also be a significant source of anxiety for autistic women. The process of building and maintaining friendships often requires a level of social intuition and spontaneity that may not come naturally. Autistic women frequently report difficulties with small talk, reading nonverbal cues, and handling the unspoken expectations that govern peer interactions.

Tony Attwood's *The Complete Guide to Asperger's Syndrome* offers insights into the nature of social interactions for autistic individuals. Attwood explains that many autistic women develop sophisticated coping strategies to navigate friendships—such as rehearsing conversation topics or mimicking the behaviors of neurotypical peers. While these strategies can lead to successful social exchanges on the surface, they also contribute to an underlying sense of dissonance. The constant effort to "keep up appearances" can be exhausting and, over time, may lead to feelings of loneliness and disconnect.

Despite these hurdles, authentic friendships are not out of reach. For many autistic women, the key to forming meaningful connections lies in finding like-minded individuals or communities that value authenticity over conformity. In online forums and support groups, for instance, many women have discovered friendships that are built on shared experiences and mutual understanding—spaces where they can set aside their masks and simply be themselves.

One story that resonates is that of Sarah (a pseudonym), who spent years feeling isolated despite having many acquaintances. It wasn't until she joined an online community dedicated to autistic women that she experienced true belonging. In that space, the nuances of her communication style were not only accepted but celebrated—a stark contrast to the expectations of broader social settings. Sarah's journey underscores the transformative power of finding one's tribe, where relationships are less about performance and more about genuine connection.

Romantic Relationships: Love, Intimacy, and Vulnerability

Romantic relationships introduce another layer of complexity. The realm of love and intimacy is fraught with expectations about emotional expression, physical affection, and social roles—all of which can be challenging for autistic women to navigate. Society often places additional pressure on women to be both emotionally available and socially adept, a combination that can be particularly taxing for someone who is managing sensory overload and communication difficulties.

In *Pretending to be Normal*, Willey recounts how the pressure to maintain a socially acceptable persona often spills over into romantic relationships. The effort to mask autistic traits can create an imbalance, where the internal emotional world remains hidden even as the external presentation appears "perfect." This disconnect can lead to misunderstandings, unmet emotional needs, and a sense of isolation within the relationship.

Yet, there are also remarkable stories of love and resilience. Many autistic women have found partners who appreciate their unique perspectives and who are willing to engage in the extra work required to understand and support them. These relationships are often built on deep mutual respect and an acknowledgment of each other's differences. As Tony Attwood suggests, successful romantic relationships for autistic individuals are less about conforming to traditional norms and more about embracing one's authentic self and finding a partner who does the same.

The journey toward intimacy often involves learning to communicate needs and boundaries in ways that are both clear and compassionate. For autistic women, this might mean explicit conversations about sensory sensitivities, the need for personal space, or preferred modes of communication. While these discussions can be daunting, they are essential for building trust and fostering genuine intimacy.

Communication Styles: The Language of Connection

At the heart of every relationship lies communication—the exchange of thoughts, feelings, and experiences. For autistic women, the act of communication is layered with complexity. The reliance on masking and the learned use of neurotypical conversational scripts often means that what is said on the surface does not always reflect the inner reality.

This gap between internal experience and external expression can lead to misunderstandings and misinterpretations.

In *The Complete Guide to Asperger's Syndrome*, Tony Attwood discusses how differences in communication are often misread as disinterest or lack of empathy. Yet, many autistic women possess a rich inner life and a deep capacity for empathy—traits that may be obscured by their socially conditioned behaviors. The challenge, then, is for both autistic women and their communication partners to bridge the gap between what is felt and what is expressed.

One strategy for improving communication is the use of direct, explicit language. Rather than relying on subtle cues or implied meanings, autistic women may benefit from—and contribute to—conversations that are straightforward and unambiguous. This approach not only reduces the likelihood of miscommunication but also empowers both parties to express their needs and desires openly.

Mindfulness and reflective practices can also enhance communication. Techniques such as journaling, meditation, or even structured conversation exercises can help autistic women better understand and articulate their emotions. Over time, these practices can lead to more authentic interactions, where both partners feel seen and heard.

The Role of Social Expectations and Stereotypes

Social expectations and stereotypes play a pervasive role in shaping relationship dynamics. Autistic women often contend with the dual burden of navigating their own unique communication challenges while also contending with external pressures to behave in traditionally "feminine" ways. These expectations can be particularly rigid in the realm of romance and friendship, where societal norms dictate how women should act, feel, and express affection.

Books like *Women and Autism Spectrum Disorder* highlight how these stereotypes can distort perceptions of autistic women. Behaviors that might be seen as a sign of emotional depth—such as sensitivity or introspection—can be misinterpreted as weakness or a lack of assertiveness. Conversely, the very coping strategies that enable autistic women to manage social situations—such as masking or rehearsing social interactions—are often overlooked or misunderstood by others.

Overcoming these stereotypes requires a collective effort. It calls for increased public awareness, better training for professionals in recognizing the diversity of autistic presentations, and a willingness on the part of society to embrace differences. When the burden of conforming to narrow social norms is lifted, relationships can become spaces of genuine exchange rather than performance.

Building a Supportive Network

While romantic relationships and friendships are important, building a broader support network is equally crucial. Many autistic women find that connecting with peers who share similar experiences provides a foundation of understanding that is hard to find in other social contexts. Whether through online communities, local support groups, or specialized social events, these networks offer a safe space for sharing, learning, and growing.

The neurodiversity movement has been instrumental in fostering communities where the focus is on celebrating differences rather than enforcing conformity. Steve Silberman's *NeuroTribes* emphasizes the value of diverse perspectives in enriching our collective experience. By participating in communities that honor neurodiversity, autistic women can build relationships based on mutual respect and shared understanding. These connections not only alleviate feelings of isolation but also provide practical advice for navigating the challenges of social interaction.

Strategies for Navigating Social Relationships

Given the unique challenges and strengths of autistic women, there are several strategies that can help improve social navigation:

- **Self-Awareness and Reflection:**
- Understanding one's own communication style, sensory needs, and emotional triggers is the first step toward building healthier relationships. Regular self-reflection—through journaling or therapy—can provide insights into personal patterns and areas for growth.
- **Education and Advocacy:**
- Empowering oneself with knowledge about autism and the female autism phenotype is essential. Resources like *Pretending to be Normal* and *The Complete Guide to Asperger's Syndrome* offer both clinical insights and personal narratives that can validate one's experiences. Armed with this knowledge, autistic women can better advocate for their needs in relationships.
- **Setting Boundaries:**
- Clear boundaries are critical in any relationship. For autistic women, who may struggle with sensory overload or emotional overwhelm, it is vital to communicate personal limits—whether that means scheduling downtime, limiting social interactions, or setting clear expectations in romantic partnerships.
- **Seeking Professional Support:**
- Therapists and counselors with experience in neurodiversity can provide valuable guidance. Whether it's learning communication skills or addressing the stress of masking, professional support can help navigate the complex emotional terrain of relationships.
- **Building Communities:**
- As noted, peer support groups and online communities offer safe spaces to connect with others who share similar experiences. These

communities can provide not only emotional support but also practical advice on everything from handling social gatherings to managing conflict in relationships.

The Future of Relationships and Social Navigation

Looking forward, there is reason to be optimistic about the evolving understanding of relationships for autistic women. As awareness grows and as more voices enter the conversation, society is gradually shifting toward a more inclusive definition of what it means to connect with others. Initiatives in education, workplace training, and mental health services are increasingly recognizing the importance of neurodiversity and are adapting their approaches to better support autistic individuals.

Innovative approaches—such as social skills training that focuses on authenticity rather than rote behavior—are emerging. These methods encourage autistic women to embrace their unique strengths while developing practical strategies for social interaction. By moving away from a one-size-fits-all model of "normal" behavior, these programs are paving the way for more meaningful and fulfilling relationships.

Conclusion

Relationships and social navigation for autistic women are complex, multifaceted journeys marked by both challenges and profound opportunities for growth. From the early lessons learned in family dynamics to the nuanced dance of friendships and romantic connections, every interaction is shaped by a delicate interplay of internal experiences and external expectations.

Influential works such as *Pretending to be Normal*, *The Complete Guide to Asperger's Syndrome*, and *NeuroTribes* have shed light on the hidden struggles and overlooked strengths of autistic women in their social lives.

These narratives not only validate personal experiences but also provide a roadmap for navigating a world that often demands conformity at the expense of authenticity.

As we look to the future, the promise of more inclusive and understanding relationships is on the horizon. With greater awareness, better diagnostic tools, and more supportive communities, autistic women are increasingly empowered to forge connections that honor their true selves. By embracing neurodiversity in all its forms, society can foster relationships that are based on genuine understanding, mutual respect, and shared humanity.

Ultimately, the journey toward building and maintaining relationships is not just about social success—it is about reclaiming one's identity, finding belonging, and celebrating the unique perspectives that each individual brings to the world. In this pursuit, every conversation, every friendship, and every act of self-advocacy becomes a testament to the resilience and strength of autistic women everywhere.

This chapter has explored the intricate world of relationships and social navigation, revealing how family dynamics, friendships, and romantic connections are uniquely experienced by autistic women. By examining the interplay of masking, social expectations, and personal authenticity, we gain deeper insight into both the challenges and the profound opportunities for genuine connection. As the dialogue around neurodiversity continues to evolve, so too does the promise of relationships where every autistic woman can feel seen, understood, and valued for who she truly is.

8

Mental Health and Emotional Well-Being

The intersection of mental health and autism in women is a complex landscape, where internal experiences often diverge dramatically from external appearances. In this chapter, we explore the emotional world of autistic women—examining the prevalence of anxiety, depression, and burnout, as well as the coping mechanisms and strategies that can support well-being. Drawing upon personal narratives, clinical research, and influential works such as Liane Holliday Willey's Pretending to be Normal: Living with Asperger's Syndrome, Tony Attwood's The Complete Guide to Asperger's Syndrome, and Steve Silberman's NeuroTribes: The Legacy of Autism, we shed light on the internal struggles many autistic women face and offer insights into the pathways toward healing and self-acceptance.

The Internal Landscape: Recognizing the Emotional Toll

Autistic women often navigate a world where the pressure to conform is relentless. From early childhood, many are taught to mask their natural tendencies in order to fit societal expectations. Over time, this constant effort to "perform" normalcy can lead to a state of chronic stress. While the external world may see an individual who appears well-adjusted and socially competent, the internal experience is often marked by intense anxiety, overwhelming sensory input, and a persistent feeling of isolation.

Liane Holliday Willey's *Pretending to be Normal* recounts her own journey of battling internal turmoil while outwardly appearing to adapt seamlessly to social situations. The constant energy spent on masking—suppressing stimming behaviors, rehearsing social interactions, and meticulously monitoring emotional responses—can eventually lead to what many describe as "emotional burnout." This burnout is not simply physical exhaustion, but an erosion of the self—a depletion of the inner resources needed to sustain authenticity and joy.

The Prevalence of Anxiety and Depression

A significant body of research and countless personal testimonies point to the high prevalence of anxiety and depression among autistic women. The factors contributing to these mental health challenges are multifaceted:

- **Masking and Chronic Stress:** As explored in previous chapters, the ongoing effort to camouflage autistic traits results in persistent psychological strain. This strain is a major contributor to anxiety. The constant vigilance required to avoid social missteps or sensory overload creates a baseline of stress that can be both debilitating and exhausting.
- **Sensory Overload:** Many autistic women experience sensory sensitivities that can lead to feelings of overwhelm in everyday environments. The inability to control or predict sensory input—whether it be from bright lights, loud noises, or crowded spaces—can trigger intense anxiety and contribute to feelings of depression.

- **Social Isolation:** The internal disconnect between one's true self and the persona presented to the world often results in profound loneliness. When efforts to fit in lead to superficial relationships and the absence of genuine understanding, the risk for depression increases.

Tony Attwood, in *The Complete Guide to Asperger's Syndrome*, notes that many autistic individuals, particularly women, internalize their struggles. Rather than externalizing distress, they may experience deep-seated feelings of inadequacy, leading to depression. These emotional challenges are compounded by a lack of targeted mental health support, as traditional therapeutic approaches are often based on neurotypical frameworks that fail to address the unique needs of autistic women.

The Role of Self-Care and Therapeutic Interventions

The path toward improved mental health and emotional well-being for autistic women lies in a combination of self-care practices, professional interventions, and community support. Developing a personalized self-care regimen is crucial in mitigating the effects of chronic stress and preventing burnout. Here are several strategies that can empower autistic women to reclaim their emotional well-being:

Developing a Tailored Self-Care Routine

- **Mindfulness and Meditation:**
- Engaging in mindfulness practices can help create a sense of calm amidst the chaos of sensory overload. Techniques such as guided meditation, deep breathing exercises, and mindful movement (like yoga) have been shown to reduce anxiety and improve overall emotional regulation. These practices help in cultivating awareness

of the present moment, thereby reducing the persistent worry about social interactions and sensory triggers.

· **Sensory-Friendly Spaces:**
· Creating environments that minimize sensory overload is essential. Whether it is a quiet room with soft lighting, noise-cancelling headphones, or the use of weighted blankets, small adjustments in the environment can have a profound effect on reducing stress levels. Autistic women can benefit greatly from spaces designed to accommodate their unique sensory needs.
· **Structured Routines:**
· While flexibility is important, having a structured routine can alleviate the anxiety that comes from unpredictability. A well-planned schedule can provide a sense of control and stability, reducing the mental energy spent on planning and decision-making throughout the day.
· **Creative Outlets:**
· Engaging in creative activities—such as writing, painting, or music—offers a dual benefit. It not only serves as a mode of self-expression but also functions as a therapeutic outlet for processing complex emotions. Many autistic women find that channeling their intense inner experiences into creative projects can be both cathartic and empowering.

Therapeutic Approaches Tailored to Neurodiversity

Standard therapeutic practices are increasingly being adapted to better serve autistic women. These approaches recognize that traditional talk therapies may not always resonate with individuals whose communication styles differ from neurotypical norms. Some of the most promising interventions include:

- **Cognitive Behavioral Therapy (CBT):**
- CBT has been adapted to help autistic individuals challenge and reframe negative thought patterns. Therapists with experience in neurodiversity can guide autistic women through strategies that address the unique triggers of anxiety and depression. This form of therapy emphasizes practical problem-solving techniques while fostering self-compassion.
- **Acceptance and Commitment Therapy (ACT):**
- ACT focuses on helping individuals accept their thoughts and feelings rather than fighting them, which can be particularly effective for those who have internalized the pressures of masking. By learning to commit to actions that align with their values, autistic women can cultivate a sense of purpose and reduce the emotional toll of constant self-monitoring.
- **Mindfulness-Based Stress Reduction (MBSR):**
- MBSR programs have shown promise in reducing stress and anxiety among neurodiverse populations. These programs combine mindfulness meditation with yoga and body awareness exercises, creating a holistic approach to managing emotional dysregulation.

Peer Support and Community Engagement

Beyond individual strategies and clinical interventions, connecting with a community of peers who share similar experiences can be incredibly healing. Online forums, local support groups, and social media communities dedicated to neurodiversity provide safe spaces for autistic women to share their struggles and successes without judgment. Personal narratives—such as those found in *Pretending to be Normal* and various online memoirs—serve as both validation and inspiration.

- **Support Groups:**

- Local and online support groups offer a venue for sharing coping strategies, venting frustrations, and celebrating victories. These groups help dismantle the isolation often felt by autistic women, replacing it with a network of understanding individuals who have traversed similar paths.
- **Mentorship Programs:**
- Peer mentorship can also play a pivotal role. Connecting with someone who has navigated similar mental health challenges provides not only guidance but also hope. The knowledge that someone else has successfully managed similar issues can be incredibly reassuring and empowering.

Addressing the Stigma Surrounding Mental Health

A persistent barrier to mental well-being for many autistic women is the stigma attached to both autism and mental health challenges. Societal misconceptions often lead to internalized shame and self-doubt, further exacerbating anxiety and depression. Works like *NeuroTribes* have been instrumental in challenging these stereotypes by reframing autism as a natural variation in human neurology rather than a disorder to be cured.

Breaking down these stigmas requires a concerted effort across multiple fronts:

- **Education and Awareness:**
- Educating the public about the diverse presentations of autism can help dispel harmful myths. When society understands that the emotional struggles of autistic women are not a personal failing but a consequence of systemic barriers and unmet needs, the stigma begins to fade.
- **Advocacy:**
- Advocacy efforts, led by autistic individuals and allies, are crucial in

driving policy changes that support mental health services tailored to neurodiversity. These efforts include pushing for better training for mental health professionals, more inclusive educational policies, and increased funding for research into neurodiverse mental health.

· **Media Representation:**
· Positive and accurate representations of autistic women in media can also shift public perceptions. When television shows, films, and books portray the emotional lives of autistic women with nuance and empathy, they contribute to a broader understanding of neurodiversity and mental health.

Personal Stories: The Transformative Power of Self-Acceptance

Amid the challenges, there are countless stories of resilience and transformation. Many autistic women have found that the journey to mental well-being is intertwined with the process of self-discovery and self-acceptance. For instance, Sarah (a pseudonym) described her experience of transitioning from constant masking to embracing her authentic self as a turning point that significantly improved her mental health. Through therapy, mindfulness practices, and the support of an online community, she gradually learned to let go of the need to conform and instead focused on nurturing her inner world.

Such stories are echoed in the pages of *Pretending to be Normal*, where personal narratives provide not only validation but also practical insights into coping strategies. They remind us that while the path to mental health may be fraught with challenges, it is also filled with opportunities for growth, healing, and empowerment.

Integrating Self-Care into Daily Life

Sustainable mental health practices are those that can be woven into the fabric of daily living. For autistic women, this integration often involves creating routines that honor their sensory and emotional needs without overwhelming them. Some practical steps include:

- **Establishing Regular Downtime:**
- Carving out time each day for quiet reflection or sensory decompression—whether through reading, listening to calming music, or simply sitting in a quiet room—can help recharge emotional batteries.
- **Physical Activity:**
- Engaging in regular physical exercise, tailored to one's abilities and interests, not only improves physical health but also reduces stress. Activities like walking, swimming, or even dancing can serve as both a physical outlet and a way to boost mood.
- **Nutrition and Sleep:**
- A balanced diet and sufficient sleep are foundational to good mental health. For many autistic women, establishing routines around mealtimes and bedtime can provide a sense of stability that supports overall well-being.
- **Creative Expression:**
- Whether it's journaling, painting, or playing an instrument, creative outlets offer a way to process complex emotions. These activities can serve as both a form of therapy and a means to communicate experiences that are difficult to articulate verbally.

The Future of Mental Health Support for Autistic Women

As our understanding of the unique mental health needs of autistic women evolves, so too does the promise of better support systems. The integration of neurodiversity into mainstream mental health practices is slowly reshaping the landscape, with an increasing number of clinicians and support organizations dedicated to providing tailored services. Future directions may include:

- **Specialized Training Programs:**
- Mental health professionals are beginning to receive training on the nuances of autism in women, which promises to improve the accuracy of diagnoses and the effectiveness of therapeutic interventions.
- **Community-Based Programs:**
- Grassroots initiatives that focus on building supportive communities can complement clinical services. These programs empower autistic women to take charge of their mental health through peer-led workshops, mindfulness sessions, and creative groups.
- **Research and Innovation:**
- Ongoing research into the intersection of autism and mental health will continue to inform new therapeutic approaches. The contributions of works like *NeuroTribes* have already laid the groundwork for a more compassionate and scientifically informed approach to neurodiverse mental health.

Conclusion

The journey toward mental health and emotional well-being for autistic women is both deeply personal and profoundly transformative. By acknowledging the intense internal challenges—ranging from chronic anxiety and depression to the emotional toll of masking—we can begin to create pathways for healing that honor the unique experiences of neurodiverse individuals. Drawing on insights from influential works such as *Pretending to be Normal*, *The Complete Guide to Asperger's Syndrome*, and *NeuroTribes*, we recognize that the struggle for mental health is not a sign of weakness but a call to build systems of support that are as diverse and resilient as the women they serve.

Through tailored self-care practices, innovative therapeutic interventions, and the power of community, autistic women are discovering ways to reclaim their emotional landscapes. Their stories of resilience, transformation, and self-acceptance illuminate a future where mental health is not defined by the pressures to conform, but by the courage to embrace one's authentic self.

As society continues to evolve toward a more inclusive understanding of neurodiversity, the promise of improved mental health support becomes ever more tangible. With continued advocacy, research, and compassionate care, the mental health journey for autistic women can shift from one of struggle and isolation to one of empowerment, resilience, and profound self-discovery.

This chapter has traversed the intricate terrain of mental health and emotional well-being for autistic women, uncovering the interplay between chronic stress, sensory overload, and the pervasive impact of masking. By integrating clinical insights, personal narratives, and the wisdom found in seminal works like *Pretending to be Normal*, *The Complete Guide to Asperger's Syndrome*, and *NeuroTribes*, we gain a comprehensive understanding of the challenges—and the opportunities—for healing in a neurodiverse world.

In embracing the full spectrum of their emotional experiences, autistic women not only validate their struggles but also chart a course toward a more authentic, fulfilling life. The journey is not easy, but it is marked by incremental breakthroughs and the enduring power of self-acceptance.

With each step, a brighter future emerges—one where mental health is recognized as a vital component of overall well-being, and where the unique needs of neurodiverse women are met with empathy, innovation, and unwavering support.

9

Building a Supportive Community

Building a supportive community is essential to the well-being and empowerment of autistic women. For far too long, many have felt isolated and misunderstood—not only by society at large but also within the systems that are meant to offer help. In this chapter, we explore the importance of cultivating networks that validate and celebrate neurodiversity. We delve into the ways in which autistic women can forge meaningful connections with peers, family, and professionals, and how these networks can become a cornerstone for resilience, personal growth, and advocacy.

The Power of Belonging

A sense of belonging is a fundamental human need. For autistic women, this need is often complicated by a history of social misunderstanding and misdiagnosis. Many have spent years feeling different and disconnected due to the pressures of masking and the relentless pursuit of conforming to neurotypical standards. Yet, it is in communities that share common experiences—where differences are not only accepted but celebrated—that true healing and empowerment can occur.

Being part of a supportive community provides a safe space where one can share personal narratives, validate internal experiences, and access a wealth of knowledge from those who truly understand the nuances of the autistic experience. These communities not only offer emotional sustenance but also practical guidance for navigating life's myriad challenges, from managing sensory overload to advocating for accommodations in the workplace.

Creating Connections: From Isolation to Integration

Historically, the societal narrative around autism has often painted a picture of isolation. Autistic women, in particular, have been marginalized by research and clinical practices that focus predominantly on male presentations of the condition. This skewed understanding has left many feeling as though their experiences do not matter or are not worthy of validation. However, the tide is slowly turning as more voices call for inclusivity and a broader understanding of neurodiversity.

One of the most transformative shifts has been the rise of online platforms and social media groups. These virtual communities have become invaluable for autistic women seeking connection, offering forums where individuals can share their stories, exchange advice, and build lasting friendships. Unlike traditional social settings where subtle differences can be overlooked or misunderstood, these online spaces are intentionally designed to be empathetic, flexible, and non-judgmental.

For example, many women have shared on platforms such as Facebook groups, Reddit threads, and specialized online forums that they finally felt seen for the first time after joining communities that celebrate neurodiversity. The shared language, experiences, and challenges create a common ground that transcends geographical boundaries, making it possible for individuals to connect with others who truly "get it."

Family as the First Support Network

While peer communities offer invaluable support, the role of family in nurturing an autistic woman's sense of belonging cannot be understated. Families can be both a source of strength and a challenge, depending on the level of understanding and acceptance within the household. For many autistic women, early life experiences were marked by a lack of recognition of their unique needs. This oversight, as described in memoirs like *Pretending to be Normal*, often led to feelings of alienation and a prolonged struggle with self-identity.

Educating family members about the nuances of autism in women is a crucial step in building a supportive environment. When family members—parents, siblings, and even extended relatives—make an effort to understand the challenges and strengths associated with the female autism phenotype, they lay the groundwork for a nurturing support system. Books such as *Women and Autism Spectrum Disorder* have been instrumental in helping families reframe their perspectives, moving away from misconceptions and toward a more informed, compassionate view.

Family support can manifest in many ways: open conversations about emotional well-being, adapting home environments to be sensory-friendly, or even simply affirming the authenticity of the individual's experience. When families embrace neurodiversity, they not only validate the autistic woman's identity but also empower her to advocate for herself in other areas of life.

Professional Networks and Advocacy Groups

Beyond personal and family circles, professional networks and advocacy groups play a critical role in shaping a more inclusive society. These organizations work to educate, influence policy, and provide direct support to autistic individuals and their families. Advocacy groups have been at the forefront of challenging outdated diagnostic criteria and pushing for changes in educational and workplace practices.

Professional networks that focus on neurodiversity in the workplace, for example, offer training sessions and workshops designed to create more accommodating environments. These initiatives not only benefit autistic women by creating safer, more understanding spaces but also benefit organizations by harnessing diverse talents and perspectives. As Tony Attwood emphasizes in *The Complete Guide to Asperger's Syndrome*, recognizing and accommodating neurodiverse individuals is not merely an act of compassion—it is also a catalyst for innovation and progress.

Similarly, mental health professionals who specialize in neurodiversity provide tailored services that are sensitive to the unique experiences of autistic women. These professionals can serve as vital connectors, linking individuals with resources such as support groups, educational programs, and therapeutic interventions. Their expertise helps demystify the complex interplay between autism and mental health, offering strategies to manage anxiety, depression, and the emotional toll of masking.

Cultivating Safe Spaces

Creating safe spaces—both physical and virtual—is a key component of building a supportive community. Safe spaces are environments where autistic women can drop their masks, express themselves authentically, and engage with others without the fear of judgment or misunderstanding. These spaces can be found in various forms:

- **Online Communities:** Virtual forums and social media groups provide immediate access to peers who share similar experiences. The anonymity and flexibility of online interactions can make it easier for individuals to open up and share their stories.

- **Local Support Groups:** In-person meetings, whether held at community centers, libraries, or local advocacy organizations, offer the opportunity for face-to-face interaction. These groups often include a blend of autistic individuals, family members, and professionals who together create a multi-dimensional support system.
- **Specialized Workshops and Retreats:** Events focused on self-care, mindfulness, or vocational training provide both educational content and a space for meaningful connection. These gatherings can help individuals build skills while also deepening their sense of community.

The emphasis in these safe spaces is on empathy, understanding, and shared experience. Rather than forcing autistic women to conform to neurotypical norms, these environments honor their unique ways of being and foster a sense of pride in neurodiversity.

The Role of Peer Mentorship

Peer mentorship is an invaluable component of supportive communities. Connecting with someone who has navigated similar challenges provides not only practical advice but also emotional reassurance. Mentors can offer insights into managing everyday challenges, navigating social interactions, and balancing the demands of work and life—all from the perspective of someone who truly understands.

Mentorship programs specifically designed for autistic women have emerged in recent years, often facilitated by advocacy groups or online communities. These programs pair experienced mentors with individuals who are new to the community or struggling to find their footing. The relationships that develop are often characterized by mutual respect, shared empathy, and a deep sense of connection that transcends traditional hierarchical structures.

The impact of peer mentorship is profound. It creates a ripple effect—empowered individuals go on to become mentors themselves, fostering a continuous cycle of support and empowerment that strengthens the entire community.

Overcoming Barriers: From Isolation to Empowerment

Despite the many benefits of supportive communities, barriers to connection still exist. Social stigma, internalized shame, and past experiences of rejection can all impede the process of building new relationships. For many autistic women, the prospect of reaching out and forming meaningful connections is daunting, particularly after years of feeling misunderstood or invalidated.

One of the first steps in overcoming these barriers is self-acceptance. Recognizing that one's experiences and ways of being are valid is essential to forming healthy relationships. Books like *Pretending to be Normal* and *NeuroTribes* have played a crucial role in reshaping the narrative around autism, encouraging individuals to view their differences not as deficits, but as strengths. This shift in perspective is foundational—it paves the way for seeking out and embracing communities that value authenticity over conformity.

Therapeutic support can also help in overcoming the internal barriers to community building. Therapists who specialize in neurodiversity can guide autistic women through the process of building self-esteem, addressing past traumas, and developing communication strategies that honor their unique needs. These interventions are most effective when integrated with community support, creating a holistic framework for personal growth.

The Ripple Effect: How Supportive Communities Change Society

The impact of building a supportive community extends far beyond the individual—it has the potential to reshape societal attitudes and practices. As more autistic women find their voice and share their experiences, they challenge the narrow definitions of what it means to be "normal." This collective empowerment fosters a broader cultural shift, one that values diversity, inclusivity, and the contributions of every individual.

Advocacy efforts, fueled by the strength of supportive communities, are driving changes in education, healthcare, and employment. Schools are beginning to adopt more flexible curricula and teaching methods that accommodate diverse learning styles. Workplaces are implementing policies that support sensory needs and promote flexible working conditions. Healthcare professionals are receiving training to better understand and serve neurodiverse populations. These changes, while incremental, represent a significant step toward a more inclusive society where every individual has the opportunity to thrive.

Moreover, as supportive communities continue to grow, they become a powerful force for advocacy. Collective voices—sharing stories, highlighting successes, and calling out systemic shortcomings—can influence public policy and drive meaningful reform. The evolution of the neurodiversity movement is a testament to this power; what began as isolated pockets of support have now blossomed into a global call for recognition, acceptance, and respect.

Practical Steps for Building Your Own Community

For those looking to cultivate a supportive community, here are some practical steps to get started:

- **Reach Out:**
- Begin by connecting with local or online groups focused on neurodiversity. Platforms like Facebook, Meetup, and specialized forums provide a wealth of options.
- **Attend Events:**
- Participate in workshops, support group meetings, or community events. In-person interactions can be transformative and help solidify virtual connections.
- **Share Your Story:**
- Embrace vulnerability by sharing your experiences, either through writing, social media, or conversations. Authentic storytelling not only validates your experience but also encourages others to open up.
- **Offer Support:**
- As you build connections, remember that community is reciprocal. Offering your support, advice, or a listening ear can strengthen bonds and empower others.
- **Advocate for Change:**
- Use your voice to advocate for better resources, policies, and understanding within your community. Whether through volunteering or engaging in public discourse, every effort contributes to broader societal change.

The Vision of a Connected Future

Imagining a future where every autistic woman feels seen, understood, and supported is a powerful vision. It is a future where communities— both physical and virtual—serve as safe havens, enabling individuals to flourish without the constant pressure to mask or conform. In such a future, the barriers that once isolated autistic women will be replaced by networks of empathy, shared understanding, and collective strength.

This vision is already taking shape. With the increasing visibility of neurodiversity advocates, the growing number of specialized support groups, and the shift in public discourse around mental health and inclusion, there is every reason to be optimistic. The journey toward building a truly supportive community is ongoing, but each step forward represents a victory—not only for individual well-being but for the collective advancement of society.

Conclusion

Building a supportive community is more than just forming connections— it is an act of resistance against the isolation and misunderstanding that have long plagued autistic women. It is a declaration that every unique experience, every nuanced trait, and every personal struggle is worthy of recognition and celebration. By coming together—through family, peers, professional networks, and advocacy groups—autistic women can create a tapestry of support that empowers them to live authentically and thrive in a world that increasingly values neurodiversity.

As we continue to explore the full spectrum of the autistic experience, it becomes clear that no one should have to face the challenges of masking, isolation, or misunderstanding alone. The power of a supportive community lies in its ability to transform lives, provide practical guidance, and ignite a cultural shift toward true inclusion.

In embracing community, we not only uplift individual voices but also contribute to a larger movement that redefines what it means to be different. Together, we pave the way for a future where every autistic woman finds not only the support she needs but also the opportunity to lead a life that is as vibrant, authentic, and empowered as she deserves.

This chapter has examined the profound impact that building a supportive community can have on the lives of autistic women. By transitioning from isolation to connection, fostering safe spaces, and championing peer mentorship and advocacy, we lay the groundwork for a future where neurodiversity is celebrated and every voice is valued. The journey toward building such communities is both personal and collective—a journey that, with every connection forged, brings us closer to a world of true inclusion and empowerment.

10

Self-Advocacy and Identity Formation

Self-advocacy and identity formation lie at the heart of the journey for many autistic women. This chapter explores how embracing one's authentic self can serve as both a catalyst for personal empowerment and a pathway toward societal change. As we delve into the processes of self-discovery, assertiveness, and the redefinition of what it means to be autistic, we draw on a wealth of personal narratives, clinical insights, and influential works in the field such as Pretending to be Normal: Living with Asperger's Syndrome by Liane Holliday Willey, The Complete Guide to Asperger's Syndrome by Tony Attwood, and NeuroTribes: The Legacy of Autism by Steve Silberman.

Embracing the Authentic Self

For many autistic women, the struggle to form an authentic identity begins early in life. From a young age, societal expectations and the necessity of masking—adopting behaviors to fit in—force many to internalize a version of themselves that is not entirely their own. This early conflict often leads to an identity divided between a public persona and a private inner world that remains unexpressed. Over time, however, the journey toward self-advocacy becomes a means of reconciling these parts and forging an identity rooted in truth and self-acceptance.

Liane Holliday Willey's *Pretending to be Normal* poignantly illustrates this conflict, describing how the pressure to conform can obscure the very qualities that make one unique. The realization that the strategies of masking, though useful in navigating social environments, are unsustainable in the long run is often a turning point. It is in the process of unmasking—of daring to let one's true self be seen—that the foundation for genuine self-advocacy is built.

The Process of Self-Discovery

Self-discovery is a gradual process that involves exploring personal strengths, weaknesses, passions, and challenges. For autistic women, this journey is frequently marked by periods of introspection and reflection. It may begin with a recognition of the discrepancies between how they feel internally and how they are expected to behave externally.

Reflective Practices

Techniques such as journaling, mindfulness, and meditation have been repeatedly recommended by therapists and peers alike. These practices allow individuals to examine their inner thoughts and feelings without judgment. By regularly reflecting on personal experiences, many autistic women learn to identify triggers for stress and anxiety, as well as moments of joy and clarity. Over time, this self-awareness forms the bedrock upon which a more authentic identity can be constructed.

For example, journaling not only provides an outlet for emotional expression but also serves as a historical record of one's evolving self. In *The Complete Guide to Asperger's Syndrome*, Tony Attwood underscores the importance of recognizing personal patterns—both in behavior and thought. This recognition can empower autistic women to challenge internalized negative messages and to celebrate their inherent strengths.

Challenging Stereotypes and Internalized Beliefs

A significant hurdle in identity formation is the internalization of societal stereotypes. Autistic women are often bombarded with messages that devalue neurodiversity, suggesting that traits such as intense focus, sensitivity, or a preference for solitude are deficiencies rather than differences. Overcoming these harmful narratives requires a deliberate and conscious effort to reframe one's self-concept.

The neurodiversity movement, as articulated in Steve Silberman's *NeuroTribes*, provides an empowering alternative to deficit-based models of autism. This perspective champions the idea that neurological differences are natural variations, not disorders to be fixed. By adopting this viewpoint, autistic women can begin to see their traits as integral components of a rich, diverse identity. This paradigm shift is not merely academic—it resonates on a deeply personal level, enabling individuals to embrace their authentic selves without shame.

Strategies for Self-Advocacy

Self-advocacy involves both understanding one's rights and communicating one's needs effectively. It is a dynamic process that evolves as individuals gain greater insight into their own identities and the environments in which they live. For many autistic women, the transition from masking to self-advocacy represents a reclaiming of personal agency.

Learning to Speak Up

One of the first steps in self-advocacy is learning to speak up about one's needs and boundaries. This might involve simple, everyday interactions—such as requesting accommodations in a workplace or clarifying sensory preferences in social settings. Effective self-advocacy requires not only self-awareness but also the development of communication skills that can bridge the gap between internal experiences and external expectations.

Training programs, workshops, and peer-led support groups can be invaluable in this regard. Many autistic women have found that learning from mentors who have successfully navigated the challenges of self-advocacy provides both practical tools and emotional reassurance. In many communities, the act of speaking up becomes not just a personal milestone, but also an act of resistance against the stigmatization of neurodiversity.

Navigating Institutional Systems

Self-advocacy also extends to interactions with institutional systems such as schools, workplaces, and healthcare services. In these settings, autistic women often face the additional challenge of having to educate others about their needs. For example, requesting specific accommodations—whether they pertain to sensory sensitivities, communication styles, or scheduling flexibility—requires a level of assertiveness that may not come naturally to someone who has long been conditioned to mask.

The work of advocacy groups and legal protections, such as the Americans with Disabilities Act (ADA) in the United States or similar legislation in other countries, plays a critical role in supporting self-advocacy. These frameworks not only provide a legal basis for requesting accommodations but also validate the experiences of autistic individuals. Engaging with these systems—through self-advocacy training or by joining advocacy networks—can empower autistic women to effect meaningful change both for themselves and for the broader community.

Building a Personal Support Network

Another vital aspect of self-advocacy is the establishment of a personal support network. This network can consist of family, friends, therapists, mentors, and peers who understand and respect the individual's experiences. In these circles, autistic women can practice self-expression without the fear of judgment, receive constructive feedback, and gain the confidence needed to advocate for themselves in more challenging environments.

Support networks are often fostered within specialized communities and online groups dedicated to neurodiversity. The mutual exchange of experiences and strategies helps individuals learn not only how to articulate their own needs but also how to navigate complex social and institutional landscapes. Such communities serve as a reminder that self-advocacy is not an isolated endeavor—it is a collective process that benefits from shared wisdom and solidarity.

The Intersection of Identity and Advocacy

Self-advocacy and identity formation are deeply intertwined. As autistic women come to understand and embrace their authentic selves, they naturally become more effective advocates for their own needs. This transformation is both personal and political, challenging the prevailing narratives that have long marginalized neurodiverse voices.

Celebrating Neurodiversity

A critical component of identity formation is the celebration of neurodiversity. By viewing autism as a natural variation rather than a
deficiency, autistic women can begin to appreciate the unique strengths
that come with their neurological makeup. Attributes such as intense
focus, creative problem-solving, and deep empathy are reinterpreted
not as deficits but as valuable contributions to society.

This shift in perspective is central to the ethos of the neurodiversity
movement. As discussed in *NeuroTribes*, embracing neurological differences fosters a more inclusive and innovative society—one in which
diversity is seen as a source of strength. For many autistic women, this
celebration of difference is a powerful antidote to years of self-doubt
and internalized stigma. It transforms the narrative from one of struggle
and inadequacy to one of empowerment and pride.

Crafting an Authentic Narrative

Another important aspect of identity formation is the creation of an
authentic personal narrative. Many autistic women have spent years
trying to fit into molds that do not align with their true selves. The
process of writing one's own story—whether through memoir, art, or
public speaking—can be a liberating experience that reclaims control
over one's identity.

In sharing their journeys, individuals not only validate their own
experiences but also provide a roadmap for others who are navigating
similar challenges. Personal narratives have the power to reshape public
perceptions and to dismantle harmful stereotypes. They serve as a
reminder that the diversity of human experience is a strength to be
celebrated rather than a problem to be fixed.

The Role of Creative Expression

Creative expression is often a powerful tool for both self-advocacy and identity formation. Many autistic women find that artistic endeavors—such as writing, painting, music, or dance—offer a means to communicate aspects of their inner world that are difficult to articulate through conventional language. These creative outlets can help bridge the gap between internal experiences and external expression, allowing individuals to share their authentic selves in a way that resonates with others.

Creative expression also fosters a sense of community. When individuals share their work, they create opportunities for connection and dialogue, challenging the notion that differences must be hidden away. Instead, creative works become a platform for advocacy, sparking conversations about neurodiversity and encouraging others to embrace their own unique identities.

The Impact of Self-Advocacy on Personal and Social Change

The journey toward self-advocacy and authentic identity formation is not only transformative on a personal level—it also has far-reaching social implications. As more autistic women learn to advocate for themselves, they contribute to a broader cultural shift that redefines what it means to be neurodiverse. Their voices challenge long-standing stereotypes and inspire changes in policy, education, and public discourse.

Through self-advocacy, autistic women are increasingly shaping conversations around mental health, employment, and accessibility. Their efforts lead to more inclusive environments in schools and workplaces, improved access to tailored healthcare, and a deeper societal understanding of neurodiversity. Each act of self-advocacy—no matter how small—serves as a building block for systemic change, paving the way for a future where every individual's unique experiences are recognized and valued.

Overcoming Barriers and Sustaining Empowerment

Despite the progress made in self-advocacy, many challenges remain. Barriers such as societal stigma, internalized self-doubt, and institutional rigidity continue to pose obstacles. However, the very act of confronting these challenges often reinforces an individual's resolve. Self-advocacy is not a destination but an ongoing process—one that requires continual learning, adaptation, and resilience.

Support networks, professional mentorship, and community advocacy are critical in helping individuals sustain their empowerment over time. Continuous education about neurodiversity and the sharing of success stories further strengthen the collective movement toward inclusivity. For autistic women, each step taken to assert their rights and express their true selves contributes to a legacy of empowerment for future generations.

Conclusion

The journey of self-advocacy and identity formation is a transformative process that lies at the core of the autistic experience for many women. It is a path marked by introspection, resilience, and the courageous decision to embrace one's authentic self in the face of societal pressures to conform. By learning to speak up, challenging internalized stereotypes, and celebrating neurodiversity, autistic women not only empower themselves but also help to reshape the broader cultural narrative.

Influential works such as *Pretending to be Normal*, *The Complete Guide to Asperger's Syndrome*, and *NeuroTribes* have illuminated the complexities of this journey, offering insights and inspiration to those navigating the challenges of identity formation. As individuals craft authentic narratives and forge supportive networks, they create ripples of change that extend far beyond personal well-being—contributing to a society that recognizes and values every form of human difference.

In the end, self-advocacy is both a deeply personal act and a powerful tool for social change. It transforms the internal struggles of masking and self-doubt into a collective call for recognition, acceptance, and respect. With every story shared and every boundary set, a new chapter of empowerment is written—one that honors the unique strengths and perspectives of autistic women and paves the way for a more inclusive future.

This chapter has explored the multifaceted process of self-advocacy and identity formation, highlighting the importance of embracing one's authentic self and challenging the societal norms that have long obscured the true beauty of neurodiversity. Through reflective practices, creative expression, and the cultivation of supportive networks, autistic women are forging paths that not only uplift their own lives but also contribute to a broader movement for change. As each voice rises in the call for acceptance and empowerment, the vision of a society where every individual is valued for who they truly are becomes ever more attainable.

11

Strategies for Daily Living and Career Success

Living life fully while navigating the challenges of autism often requires developing specialized strategies for daily living and career success. Autistic women face a unique set of obstacles—from managing sensory overload and executive functioning to overcoming social and workplace challenges—that can make daily tasks and professional advancement particularly daunting. This chapter offers a comprehensive guide to practical tools, adaptive strategies, and actionable advice for thriving both at home and in the workplace. Drawing on insights from influential works such as Liane Holliday Willey's Pretending to be Normal: Living with Asperger's Syndrome, Tony Attwood's The Complete Guide to Asperger's Syndrome, and Steve Silberman's NeuroTribes: The Legacy of Autism, we explore methods to organize daily routines, manage stress, and build a fulfilling career that honors one's unique strengths.

Mastering Daily Life: Tools for Practical Living

Establishing a Structured Routine

A well-planned daily routine can alleviate the mental energy required for decision-making and provide a sense of stability. For many autistic women, unpredictability can trigger anxiety and sensory overwhelm. Here are key elements to consider when building your routine:

- **Morning Rituals:** Start your day with a consistent wake-up routine that includes time for self-care, such as a calming cup of tea or a short mindfulness exercise. Establishing a morning ritual sets a positive tone for the day.
- **Visual Schedules:** Visual calendars, planners, or apps designed for time management can be extremely useful. By breaking the day into clear segments, you can better manage tasks and reduce uncertainty. Tony Attwood's work emphasizes that clear, concrete schedules help in reducing executive function challenges that many autistic individuals experience.
- **Buffer Times:** Build short breaks between tasks. These buffer periods help prevent the accumulation of stress and provide a moment to recalibrate if sensory overload or fatigue begins to set in.

Managing Sensory Overload and Stress

Daily living often involves navigating environments that may be over-whelming due to sensory input. Here are strategies to maintain calm in sensory-rich settings:

- **Designated Quiet Spaces:** Create a personal sanctuary at home where you can retreat to decompress. This might include soft lighting, comfortable seating, and noise-cancelling headphones.
- **Sensory Tools:** Experiment with sensory aids like weighted blankets,

fidget tools, or aromatherapy. These tools, mentioned in various neurodiversity resources, can help regulate sensory inputs and provide comfort during stressful times.

- **Mindfulness and Relaxation Techniques:** Integrating mindfulness practices such as deep breathing, progressive muscle relaxation, or meditation into your routine can reduce anxiety and promote emotional regulation. Resources like *Pretending to be Normal* provide practical advice on mindfulness techniques that have helped many navigate daily challenges.

Organizational Strategies

Executive functioning challenges can make tasks like time management, planning, and organization more difficult. Consider the following strategies:

- **Task Lists:** Use checklists to break down larger tasks into manageable steps. This method reduces cognitive overload and helps maintain focus.
- **Digital Tools:** Productivity apps like calendars, reminders, and to-do lists (e.g., Trello, Todoist, or even simple smartphone reminders) can be invaluable for staying organized and tracking progress.
- **Environmental Cues:** Utilize labels, color-coded systems, or sticky notes around the home to provide visual prompts for tasks and routines. Such cues can serve as gentle reminders and help maintain an orderly environment.

Career Success: Navigating the Workplace with Confidence

Achieving career success while managing the nuances of autism requires both self-awareness and the development of practical workplace strategies. The workplace environment often demands quick adaptations, social interaction, and the ability to multitask—all of which can present unique challenges for autistic women.

Identifying Strengths and Interests

One of the first steps in carving out a successful career is to recognize and leverage your unique strengths:

- **Focused Interests:** Autistic women often have intense, focused interests that can translate into specialized skills or knowledge. Embrace these passions, as they can set you apart in the job market.
- **Detail Orientation:** Many autistic individuals are known for their attention to detail. Highlighting this strength can be advantageous in fields that require precision, such as data analysis, research, design, or quality assurance.
- **Creative Problem-Solving:** Creativity is a hallmark of neurodiverse thinking. Whether through innovative solutions or unconventional approaches, your ability to see problems from a unique perspective is a valuable asset.

Seeking the Right Workplace Environment

The right work environment is essential for both productivity and mental well-being. Consider the following when evaluating potential job opportunities:

- **Flexible Work Options:** Many autistic women thrive in environments that offer flexible hours, remote work, or a hybrid model. Flexibility can reduce the stress associated with long commutes and rigid schedules.
- **Sensory-Friendly Settings:** Look for workplaces that provide accommodations for sensory needs, such as quiet workspaces, adjustable lighting, or the ability to control ambient noise. Employers who understand the importance of these accommodations can make a significant difference in your work experience.
- **Inclusive Culture:** Seek out organizations that value neurodiversity and have established programs or policies to support neurodiverse employees. Companies that are proactive about inclusion and offer mentorship programs can help foster a more supportive and understanding environment.

Effective Communication and Self-Advocacy at Work

Communication is a cornerstone of career success. For autistic women, adapting communication styles in the workplace can help bridge the gap between internal experience and external expectations.

- **Clear Communication:** Practice clear and direct communication. It can be helpful to prepare in advance for meetings or presentations by outlining key points and rehearsing responses to potential questions. As Tony Attwood notes in *The Complete Guide to Asperger's Syndrome*, preparation can ease anxiety and lead to more confident interactions.
- **Requesting Accommodations:** Know your rights and the accommodations available under legislation such as the Americans with Disabilities Act (ADA) or similar laws in your country. When necessary, don't hesitate to request reasonable adjustments that can improve your work performance and reduce stress.

- **Feedback and Reflection:** Regularly seek constructive feedback from supervisors and colleagues. This practice not only demonstrates your commitment to growth but also provides insight into areas where you can further develop your skills. Additionally, reflecting on feedback helps align your communication style with workplace expectations without compromising authenticity.

Balancing Work and Self-Care

Maintaining a balance between work responsibilities and personal well-being is crucial for long-term career success. Here are strategies to manage this balance:

- **Set Clear Boundaries:** Define specific work hours and create a physical and mental separation between work and home life. For example, if you work remotely, designate a particular area of your home as your workspace.
- **Scheduled Breaks:** Incorporate regular breaks into your workday to prevent burnout. Short, scheduled periods of rest can help reset your focus and reduce the cumulative stress of long work sessions.
- **Mindful Transitions:** Use transitional activities, such as a brief walk or a short meditation session, to shift gears between tasks. These transitions can help ease the mental shift from work-related stress to personal relaxation.
- **Leverage Technology:** Consider productivity tools that remind you to take breaks, manage your time, and monitor your workload. Digital wellness tools can assist in maintaining a healthy balance, ensuring that work does not overwhelm your personal life.

Long-Term Career Development and Growth

Career success is not solely about day-to-day management—it also involves long-term planning, continuous learning, and professional growth.

Setting Career Goals

Define clear, realistic career goals that reflect both your interests and your strengths. Consider:

- **Short-Term Objectives:** Identify achievable goals for the next few months—such as mastering a new skill, improving your communication in meetings, or developing a more efficient workflow.
- **Long-Term Aspirations:** Think about where you want to be in five or ten years. Whether it's moving into a leadership role, starting your own business, or transitioning to a different field, having a vision for the future can motivate and guide your professional development.

Pursuing Professional Development

Ongoing education and training are essential for staying competitive and growing in your career:

- **Workshops and Courses:** Enroll in professional development courses that align with your interests. Many community colleges, online platforms, and professional organizations offer courses that can enhance your skills in areas such as technology, management, or creative arts.
- **Networking Opportunities:** Attend industry conferences, webinars, and networking events. These opportunities allow you to connect

with peers, learn about industry trends, and gain insights into potential career advancements.

- **Mentorship Programs:** Seek out mentorship opportunities within your organization or through professional networks. A mentor who understands the nuances of neurodiversity can offer tailored advice and help you navigate career challenges more effectively.

Leveraging Your Unique Perspective

Your neurodiverse perspective is not just a personal characteristic—it can be a competitive advantage in the workplace. Embrace your ability to think outside conventional paradigms:

- **Innovation Through Diversity:** Share your unique insights and approaches to problem-solving. Many organizations are actively seeking diverse perspectives to drive innovation and improve decision-making.
- **Documenting Success:** Keep a record of your accomplishments, projects, and the positive impact of your contributions. This documentation can be invaluable during performance reviews, salary negotiations, or when seeking new opportunities.
- **Building Your Personal Brand:** Use social media, professional networks like LinkedIn, or even personal blogs to showcase your expertise and share your journey. Building a personal brand that reflects your strengths and authentic self can open doors to new career opportunities.

Integrating Daily Living Strategies with Career Success

Success in daily living and the workplace is interconnected. When you establish effective routines at home, manage stress efficiently, and harness your unique strengths, you're better equipped to excel in your professional life. Conversely, a supportive work environment that values your contributions can reinforce positive habits at home.

Creating Synergy Between Home and Work

- **Unified Planning:** Use the same organizational tools and routines at home and in the workplace. Consistency across environments can reduce cognitive load and streamline your daily activities.
- **Transferable Skills:** Skills developed for personal time management, stress reduction, and organization can directly enhance your productivity at work. Recognizing this synergy reinforces the value of self-care in all areas of life.
- **Work-Life Integration:** Aim for integration rather than strict separation. When your work environment is flexible and understanding of your needs, it becomes easier to align your personal goals with professional responsibilities.

The Role of Self-Reflection

Regular self-reflection is a recurring theme in both daily living and career success. Evaluate what strategies work for you and where adjustments are needed:

- **Weekly Reviews:** Set aside time each week to review your accomplishments, challenges, and goals. This practice helps identify patterns, celebrate progress, and plan for future improvements.

- **Feedback Loops:** Encourage honest feedback from colleagues and mentors. Use this input to refine your strategies and ensure continuous growth.
- **Celebrate Milestones:** Recognize and reward yourself for small victories—whether it's successfully managing a challenging meeting or maintaining a balanced routine for a month. Celebrating milestones reinforces positive behavior and builds confidence.

Conclusion

Strategies for daily living and career success are essential for autistic women seeking to thrive in a world that often demands neurotypical behaviors. By establishing structured routines, managing sensory challenges, and leveraging unique strengths, you can create a balanced and fulfilling life both at home and in the workplace. Embracing clear communication, effective organization, and continuous professional development allows you to transform daily challenges into opportunities for growth.

The insights from influential works like *Pretending to be Normal*, *The Complete Guide to Asperger's Syndrome*, and *NeuroTribes* serve as guiding lights on this journey, offering practical advice and validation for your experiences. As you integrate these strategies, remember that the pursuit of balance and success is a dynamic, ongoing process—one that requires adaptation, self-compassion, and the courage to remain authentic.

Every step taken toward organizing your day, advocating for your needs, and showcasing your unique talents is a step toward a future where your contributions are valued and your well-being is prioritized. In embracing both your personal and professional aspirations, you not only enhance your own life but also contribute to a broader shift toward a more inclusive, understanding society.

Ultimately, the journey toward daily living strategies and career success is about harnessing your full potential and recognizing that your neurodiverse perspective is a powerful asset. With thoughtful planning, resilient self-care, and an unwavering commitment to authenticity, you can build a life and a career that are as vibrant and dynamic as you are.

This chapter has explored a comprehensive range of strategies designed to support everyday living and professional growth. By combining practical tools with insights from seminal works, we have laid out a roadmap that empowers autistic women to manage daily challenges, navigate complex work environments, and achieve meaningful success. Through consistency, reflection, and a commitment to leveraging your unique strengths, you can transform obstacles into opportunities and pave the way for a fulfilling future that honors your true self.

12

Looking Ahead – The Future of Understanding and Support

As we reach the final chapter, we turn our gaze toward the horizon—a future where the understanding and support of autistic women continue to evolve. The past decades have brought significant breakthroughs in recognizing the female autism phenotype, reshaping diagnostic practices, and empowering individuals to embrace their authentic selves. Today, we stand at the threshold of a new era, one where research, policy, community, and advocacy are converging to create a more inclusive and supportive environment. In this chapter, we explore emerging trends, the impact of advocacy, technological innovations, and future directions for research and support services.

Emerging Research and Evolving Perspectives

The landscape of autism research is changing rapidly. For many years, studies on autism focused primarily on male presentations of the condition. However, as the concept of the female autism phenotype gains acceptance, research is increasingly honing in on the nuances that distinguish autistic women from their male counterparts.

Recent studies are beginning to investigate the subtle differences in sensory processing, emotional regulation, and social communication that are often masked in autistic women. These studies, along with the groundbreaking work presented in *NeuroTribes: The Legacy of Autism* by Steve Silberman, are helping to refine diagnostic criteria. Researchers are also exploring the genetic, environmental, and neurological factors that contribute to the diversity of autism presentations. This emerging body of work promises not only to improve diagnostic accuracy but also to inform more effective, personalized interventions.

Moreover, interdisciplinary collaboration between psychologists, neuroscientists, and sociologists is fostering a more holistic view of autism. Integrating qualitative research—such as personal narratives and memoirs found in *Pretending to be Normal: Living with Asperger's Syndrome* by Liane Holliday Willey—with quantitative studies is creating a richer understanding of what it means to be autistic. As these diverse perspectives merge, the future holds the promise of a more inclusive and empathetic approach to neurodiversity.

Policy and Advocacy: Shaping a More Inclusive Society

The push for greater inclusion extends far beyond the laboratory. Policy reform and advocacy efforts are playing a crucial role in transforming the systems that impact autistic women. Legislative measures, like the Americans with Disabilities Act (ADA) in the United States and similar frameworks worldwide, have already provided a foundation for protecting the rights of neurodiverse individuals. However, the future demands more than just legal protections—it requires proactive policies that promote inclusion in education, employment, and healthcare.

Advocacy organizations have been instrumental in driving these changes. Groups that focus on neurodiversity and women's rights are lobbying for educational reforms, workplace accommodations, and increased funding for autism research. Their work is supported by a growing body of evidence, as outlined in influential texts like Tony Attwood's *The Complete Guide to Asperger's Syndrome*, which calls for diagnostic and support systems that recognize gender-specific nuances.

In the coming years, we can expect to see policies that not only address the current needs of autistic women but also anticipate future challenges. For instance, as technology reshapes the workplace, adaptive and flexible job environments will become increasingly critical. Policy-makers and advocacy groups are already collaborating with industries to create guidelines that promote neurodiversity as a strength—a shift that benefits everyone. With continued pressure from informed advocates and empowered communities, the future looks promising for comprehensive policy reform that honors the unique experiences of autistic women.

Technological Innovations: Tools for Empowerment and Connection

Technology is another key driver of future change. The digital revolution is providing new platforms for connection, education, and support. Online communities, telehealth services, and mobile applications are transforming the way autistic women access resources and build networks.

For many, online platforms offer a safe space to share experiences, find mentorship, and access mental health support without the pressures of in-person interactions. Social media groups, forums, and dedicated websites allow autistic women to bypass traditional barriers to communication and connect with peers from around the world. This global network of support is a testament to the resilience and adaptability of neurodiverse communities.

Moreover, telehealth has emerged as a vital resource for delivering mental health services tailored to the needs of autistic women. Remote therapy sessions, virtual support groups, and online workshops make it easier for individuals in rural or underserved areas to access specialized care. The COVID-19 pandemic accelerated these innovations, and the momentum is likely to continue, ensuring that high-quality, personalized support is available to more people than ever before.

Innovative applications are also being developed to assist with daily living and career success. For example, apps that help with scheduling, task management, and sensory regulation can be personalized to meet individual needs. These technological tools not only promote independence but also empower autistic women to thrive in both personal and professional spheres. By integrating technology with evidence-based practices, the future holds a wealth of resources designed to make everyday life more manageable and fulfilling.

Educational and Workplace Reforms: Cultivating Inclusive Environments

Education and employment are two arenas where significant improvements are on the horizon. In educational settings, there is a growing recognition of the need for individualized learning plans that accommodate diverse learning styles. Schools and universities are increasingly adopting Universal Design for Learning (UDL) principles, which offer flexible curricula and teaching methods that benefit all students, particularly those on the autism spectrum. This trend not only improves academic outcomes for autistic women but also fosters an environment of acceptance and inclusion from an early age.

Workplaces, too, are undergoing transformation. The push for diversity and inclusion is prompting companies to re-evaluate their hiring practices, workplace environments, and organizational cultures. Initiatives such as neurodiversity hiring programs and mentorship schemes are becoming more common, reflecting a broader understanding of the unique talents that autistic women bring to the table. Employers are recognizing that a workforce that values diverse perspectives is more innovative and resilient.

Future workplace policies may include enhanced sensory accommodations, flexible scheduling, and remote work options—all of which contribute to a more inclusive and supportive environment. Training programs designed to educate managers and employees about neurodiversity are also on the rise, paving the way for a corporate culture that celebrates differences rather than viewing them as obstacles. With these reforms, the future of work holds the promise of empowering autistic women to fully realize their professional potential.

The Role of Community and Peer Networks

At the heart of these advancements lies the strength of community. Support networks that have been built both online and offline are a testament to the power of shared experience and collective advocacy. Over the years, the neurodiversity movement has grown from isolated groups into a vibrant global community, uniting autistic women, their families, and allies in a common quest for understanding and support.

These communities are more than just support systems—they are hubs of innovation and empowerment. Peer mentorship programs, community-led workshops, and advocacy campaigns amplify voices that have long been marginalized. By sharing stories, challenges, and successes, autistic women not only help one another but also contribute to a broader societal shift toward acceptance and inclusion.

Looking ahead, we can expect these networks to become even more integral to the fabric of our society. As communities continue to expand and diversify, they will play a key role in shaping public policy, advancing research, and creating spaces where neurodiversity is celebrated. The ripple effect of community empowerment is profound, fostering a culture where every individual is valued for their unique contributions.

Personal Narratives: Inspiring Future Generations

The power of personal narratives cannot be overstated. Stories of resilience, struggle, and triumph have the ability to change hearts and minds. Autistic women who share their journeys provide a roadmap for future generations, illustrating that embracing one's authentic self is not only possible but also transformative.

Memoirs like *Pretending to be Normal* have long served as beacons of hope, offering both validation and inspiration to those who feel alone in their experiences. As more voices join the conversation, the collective narrative becomes richer and more diverse, challenging outdated stereotypes and inspiring others to advocate for themselves. Future generations will benefit from an ever-growing repository of stories that document the evolution of understanding and support for autistic women.

These narratives are also critical in humanizing the statistics and research findings that dominate academic discourse. They remind us that behind every study, every policy, and every technological innovation, there are real people with hopes, dreams, and unique talents. By amplifying these voices, we create a more empathetic and inclusive society—one where every autistic woman is seen, heard, and celebrated.

Future Directions for Research and Innovation

Looking ahead, the next wave of research will likely focus on further refining our understanding of the female autism phenotype. Areas of interest include the development of more sensitive diagnostic tools, the exploration of personalized interventions, and the investigation of long-term outcomes for autistic women across the lifespan. Collaborative efforts between researchers, clinicians, and community advocates will be crucial in driving these advancements.

Innovation is not limited to technology and diagnostics—it also encompasses the evolution of support services. Future initiatives may include community-based mental health programs, peer-led support networks, and comprehensive career development workshops tailored specifically for neurodiverse individuals. As our understanding deepens, so too does our ability to design interventions that are both effective and respectful of individual differences.

Interdisciplinary research that bridges the gap between science, education, and public policy will be essential. By integrating insights from fields such as neuroscience, psychology, and sociology, researchers can develop a more nuanced picture of what it means to be an autistic woman. This holistic approach will pave the way for breakthroughs that not only improve individual lives but also contribute to a broader societal transformation.

Embracing a Future of Inclusion and Empowerment

The vision for the future is one of inclusivity, where autistic women are empowered to lead fulfilling lives without the constraints of outdated stereotypes or systemic barriers. This future is built on the pillars of research, policy reform, technological innovation, and community empowerment. Each of these elements is interdependent, creating a feedback loop that drives continuous improvement.

Imagine a world where educational institutions recognize and nurture neurodiverse talents from an early age, where workplaces are designed to accommodate and celebrate differences, and where healthcare services are tailored to address the unique needs of every individual. This vision is not a distant dream—it is a tangible goal that is already being pursued through concerted advocacy and research efforts.

As society becomes more aware of the richness of neurodiversity, the barriers that once marginalized autistic women will continue to crumble. Through collective action and the relentless pursuit of understanding, the future will witness a profound shift—a move from mere tolerance to genuine celebration of human differences.

Conclusion

Looking ahead, the future of understanding and support for autistic women is bright and full of promise. Emerging research, progressive policies, technological innovations, and the power of community are converging to create a more inclusive and empathetic society. As we build on the knowledge and insights gleaned from seminal works like *NeuroTribes*, *Pretending to be Normal*, and *The Complete Guide to Asperger's Syndrome*, we move closer to a world where every autistic woman is valued, supported, and empowered.

This journey toward a more inclusive future is ongoing, driven by the resilience and determination of individuals who refuse to be defined by outdated norms. With each new breakthrough in research, each policy reform, and each personal story shared, we lay another brick in the foundation of a society that embraces neurodiversity as a strength.

In this final chapter, we celebrate not only the progress made but also the limitless potential that lies ahead. The path forward is one of collaboration, innovation, and unwavering commitment to the dignity and worth of every individual. As we look to the future, we envision a world where autistic women are not merely accommodated but are celebrated as vital contributors to the richness of human experience— a world where support, understanding, and empowerment are not privileges but rights enjoyed by all.

This chapter has charted a course for the future, highlighting emerging research, policy reforms, technological advancements, and community initiatives that promise to reshape the landscape for autistic women. As we embrace a future defined by inclusion and empowerment, every step we take brings us closer to a society where neurodiversity is not just acknowledged but celebrated. The journey continues, fueled by hope, innovation, and the collective voice of those who dare to dream of a more equitable and compassionate world.